Professional Issues in Speech-Language Pathology and Audiology

▶ Professional Issues in Speech-Language Pathology and Audiology

Franklin H. Silverman
Marquette University
Medical College of Wisconsin

Allyn and Bacon
Boston • London • Toronto • Sydney • Tokyo • Singapore

Executive Editor: Stephen D. Dragin
Editorial Assistant: Elizabeth McGuire
Editorial-Production Administrator: Joe Sweeney
Editorial-Production Service: Walsh & Associates, Inc.
Composition Buyer: Linda Cox
Manufacturing Buyer: Dave Repetto
Cover Administrator: Jennifer Hart

Library of Congress Cataloging-in-Publication Data

Silverman, Franklin H., 1933-
    Professional issues in speech-language pathology and audiology /
Franklin H. Silverman
        p.   cm.
    Includes bibliographical references.
    ISBN 0-205-27470-6
    1. Speech therapy—Practice. 2. Audiology—Practice. I. Title.
    [DNLM: 1. Speech-Language Pathology. 2. Audiology.   WL 21 S587p
1998]
    RC428.5.S55   1998
    616.85′5—dc21
    DNLM/DLC
    for Library of Congress   98-29863
                                                                          CIP

Printed in the United States of America

10   9   8   7   6   5   4   3   2   1   02   01   00   99   98

Contents

▶

Preface

A number of issues affect the management of communicative disorders and tend to be considered superficially—if at all—in the disorder-oriented courses in speech-language pathology and audiology curriculums. These are referred to in various ways, including professional issues, service delivery issues, ethical issues, legal issues, funding issues, marketing issues, and program administration issues. The American-Speech-Language-Hearing Association (ASHA) currently has as one of its priorities the acquainting of both students and practitioners with these issues and how they, as professionals, should cope with them. Evidence of ASHA's interest in alerting current and future practitioners to these issues includes devoting most of the content of its *Asha* and much of that of its *ASHA Leader* publications to them, having sessions devoted to them at its annual convention, conducting workshops dealing with them, and requiring course content in them in the training programs it accredits. Some ASHA-accredited training programs have already added a course devoted to these issues and others are likely to do so in the future.

Professional Issues in Speech-Language Pathology and Audiology is intended to acquaint students and practitioners with strategies for coping with a number of professional clinical issues. The book has several objectives. One of the main ones is to increase awareness of the need to deal appropriately with these issues in order to meet the requirement of the ASHA Code of Ethics to "hold paramount the welfare of persons served professionally." Stated somewhat differently, I am attempting to increase awareness of some ways that dealing inappropriately with these issues can cause a clinician to be out of compliance with the ASHA ethical code.

The second of my objectives is to help students and practitioners develop a more "objective attitude" toward change and increase their ability to cope with it. Regardless of whether you work in a medical or an educational setting, both your scope and manner of practice are likely to change many times during your career. Some of the changes will be both substantial and unwelcome; the current impact of the managed health-care philosophy is an example. Since change is inevitable, having an objective attitude toward it would cause you to regard the need for change as offering you a challenge rather than being a tragedy. As the old adage says, "If you are handed a lemon, make lemonade."

The third objective is to acquaint students majoring in speech-language pathology and audiology with some of the professional responsibilities and issues with which they will be expected to cope competently. The issues and responsibilities dealt with include professional ethics, credentialing, contractual aspects of the client–clinician relationship, malpractice, influencing legislation, being an expert witness, marketing clinical services, managed health care, supervising paraprofessionals, copyright considerations for clinicians, documenting treatment efficacy, patient rights, scope of practice, tax implications of employment relationships, cultural sensitivity, and facilitating report writing.

It is impossible to give credit to all the sources from which the concepts presented in this book have been drawn. This book is the result of more than thirty-five years of clinical experience with persons who have communicative disorders and of years of reading about and hundreds of hours of conversations with students and colleagues about the issues dealt with in it. Consequently, I cannot credit this or that concept to a particular person, but I can say "thank you" to all who have helped, particularly the students in my professional affairs course during the past fifteen years whose questions and criticisms have helped me to clarify my own ideas. Some special thanks are due to Dorothy Wood, Director of Marquette University's Speech Clinic and an ASHA Legislative Counselor, for her careful reading of the entire manuscript and helpful suggestions for improving it.

► 1

Introduction

In an "ideal" world:

- The only consideration in developing a management plan for a client's communicative disorder would be his or her needs.
- Whatever funding was needed would be available.
- Clients would forgive clinicians' mistakes and not sue them for malpractice.
- The bills that municipal, state, and federal legislatures consider would always be helpful—not harmful—to persons who have communicative disorders and to speech-language pathologists and audiologists as professionals.
- Clients and third-party payers would always keep their promises and consequently, written agreements (contracts) would be unnecessary.
- The level of funding available for clinical services would be adequate to make it unnecessary for some of them to be provided by paraprofessionals.
- Speech-language pathologists and audiologists would not be "strongly encouraged" by their employers to provide clinical services to persons who are highly unlikely to be helped by them for whom insurance funding is available.
- Anybody who could benefit from our services would be aware of them—that is, marketing our services to potential referral sources and the general public would be unnecessary.
- Speech-language pathologists and audiologists would always function clinically in a highly ethical manner—that is, they would always

hold paramount the welfare of the persons whom they serve professionally.
- Speech-language pathologists or audiologists would be competent to perform all of the clinical services that they are required by their employer to perform
- Clients and their families would never retain an attorney to challenge a clinician's recommendations in a court or administrative hearing.
- Speech-language pathologists and audiologists would keep their knowledge and skills up to date.
- Speech-language pathologists and audiologists would be sensitive to their clients' cultural backgrounds when interacting with them and their families and when developing plans for managing their communicative disorders.

Unfortunately, we don't live in an "ideal" world.

In the real world, considerations other than the needs of our clients and their families affect our ability to hold paramount their welfare—what the ASHA Code of Ethics declares to be our primary duty. And factors other than our own competence affect our well-being as professionals.

There is both bad and good news about societal-related considerations and factors that can adversely affect your ability to be helpful to clients and your professional well-being. The "bad news" is that they exist. The "good news" is that most can be coped with to some degree. That is, their undesirable effects on your professional well-being and on your ability to "hold paramount the welfare of the persons whom you serve professionally" can be minimized. My primary objective in this book is to provide at least some of the information that you will need to cope with them successfully.

SOCIETAL-RELATED CONSIDERATIONS AND FACTORS

Before you can develop a strategy for coping with something, you have to both be aware that it exists and understand how it can impinge on your activities. While you undoubtedly are highly aware of some of the societal-related considerations and factors that can affect your professional well-being and clinical functioning, there probably are others of which you are either unaware or have a low level of awareness. One of my goals is to increase your awareness and understanding of some of these, at least a little. Another of my goals is to assist you in developing strategies for coping with events that have the potential to adversely affect your professional well-being and your functioning as a clinician consistent with the ASHA Ethical Code. Some suggestions for doing so are provided that were gleaned from the literature and from interviews with experienced clinicians.

What types of societal-related considerations and factors can affect your professional well-being and how you manage clients' communicative disorders? To begin to answer this question, let's examine several of the "ideal world" statements with which this chapter began. One of them states that whatever funding is needed to manage a client's communicative disorder will be available for doing so—that is, the availability of funding is not a consideration for making management decisions. This is unlikely to be true for all of your clients. Those for whom it is most likely to be true are those with considerable financial resources of their own, exceptionally good medical insurance, or who are children in school systems that have exceptionally large budgets for special education services. For some persons who have communicative disorders, none of these are true. Consequently, our treatment plans for them would be likely to be influenced, at least a little, by the amount of funding available. And to provide a high quality of service to them, we may have to manage their disorders differently (but not necessarily less effectively) than we would have otherwise.

Another of these "ideal world" statements says that clients will forgive clinician's mistakes and not sue them for malpractice. While speech-language pathologists and audiologists have not been involved in malpractice litigation to the extent of practitioners in some health-related fields, they nevertheless have been sued often enough that few would work without malpractice insurance. The likelihood of speech-language pathologists becoming involved in such litigation probably will increase as a result of their assuming such new responsibilities as supervising paraprofessionals and treating serious medical conditions, such as dysphagia. To protect themselves—that is, their professional well-being—it is critical that they be aware of the legal definition of malpractice and scenarios that have resulted in speech-pathologists and audiologists becoming involved with malpractice litigation. Furthermore, they need guidelines for functioning clinically that will minimize the likelihood of their becoming involved in such litigation.

A third of these "ideal world" statements is that the bills considered and passed by municipal, state, and federal legislatures would always be helpful—not harmful—to persons who have communicative disorders and to the professional well-being of speech-language pathologists and audiologists. Perhaps the best evidence that our world is not ideal in this regard is the fact the American Speech-Language-Hearing Association utilizes both professional lobbyists and volunteers (the latter through its Congressional Action Contact Network). To meet the requirement of the ASHA Ethical Code to hold paramount the welfare of persons served professionally, it is crucial that the legislation that regulates our clinical functioning—particularly that which provides the funding for our services—be appropriate for doing so. We all have a responsibility here, even for legislation that doesn't directly affect the clients in our caseload. The persons whose welfare you are required to hold paramount include everyone in the United States who has a communicative disorder. Consequently, your responsibility to persons who are communicatively impaired extends considerably beyond the borders of your caseload. Some ways by which you can fulfill this responsibility are described in Chapter 4.

Another of these statements that is likely to be questionable is that those persons in your community who can benefit from your services are aware of them and consequently, it is unnecessary for you to market them to potential referral sources and the general public in your community. While the level of awareness of the services that we offer has certainly increased during the past twenty-five years, nevertheless many persons who could benefit from our services are still not aware of them. Evidence that supports this conclusion includes the increasing stress that the American Speech-Language-Hearing Association is placing on the need for clinicians to adequately market their clinical services (e.g., by frequently sponsoring workshops that provide information on how to do it). Obviously, we are limited in our ability to hold paramount the welfare of persons who are not aware of our services.

The impacts that these and the other considerations and factors I mentioned at the beginning of the chapter have on your professional well-being and/or on how you manage your clients' communicative disorders are explored in depth elsewhere in the book.

COPING WITH CHANGE

There is an old adage that states that the only two things in life that we can be certain of are death and taxes. Actually, there is a third—change. Nothing remains the same. As one of the ancient Greek philosophers expressed it, "You can't step in the same river twice."

While change is both normal and expected, all of us tend to resist acknowledging and accepting it to some degree. Doing so forces us to stop operating on "automatic" and switch to "manual" (at least for a short time). That is, it forces us to reevaluate the set of rules that we use to guide an aspect of our functioning. Doing so also is stressful because it implies a possible loss of control over an aspect of our world.

There are several ways that we may cope with change other than dealing with it. One is not acknowledging it—ignoring it. We would continue to cope with situations in the ways we have done so previously. The most likely consequence of our doing so is that we will be less successful in coping with them.

A second strategy that we can use to avoid dealing with change is refusing to accept it—that is, insisting on the status quo being maintained. If this is done, we can continue to operate on "automatic"—by the same set of rules. We can avoid or delay the stress that comes from having to change. Since change is normal, this strategy is highly unlikely to be successful. Consequently, the most likely outcome from using it is the same as that from using the previous one—reduced success in coping.

Change brings about a loss—a loss for which it is appropriate to grieve. The grieving process has a number of predictable stages, the first being *denial* and the last *acceptance*. While it can be beneficial psychologically immediately after experiencing a loss to *deny* that it is "real," it is highly unlikely to be so indefinitely. You need to accept the reality of the change as quickly as possible and attempt to cope it.

Speech-language pathologists and audiologists continuously experience societally induced, change-related losses with which they have to learn to cope. They appear to accept and learn to cope with most of them relatively easily. However, there are some that many appear to have a great deal of difficulty accepting and/or learning to cope with (judging, in part, by comments in ASHA journals and at ASHA "town meetings"). Two examples when this chapter was written were the widespread adoption of the "managed care" philosophy and use of paraprofessionals.

Longing for the "good old days" is normal, but not particularly helpful in coping with present realities. Our survival as a profession and our ability to continue to hold paramount the welfare of the persons whom we serve professionally will be determined, at least in part, by our ability to learn to cope with societally induced changes in the rules by which we function. While adoption of a managed care philosophy, for example, may mean that we can't continue to provide high quality care to our clients if we attempt to do it in the way we did previously, this does not necessarily mean that we can't provide our clients with high quality care. It just means that we can't do it the same way we did during the "good old days." We may, for example, have to function more in a consultative mode and/or use paraprofessionals.

How you view the need to continually change your treatment strategies because of societal changes is important. It is human nature to view it with regret. It is more comfortable to operate on "automatic" than "manual." On the other hand, being confronted by challenges to your professional survival with which you have to learn to cope can make life interesting—particularly if you are successful in coping with them most of the time!

▶ 2

Professional Ethics—Holding Paramount the Welfare of Persons Served Professionally

One of the societal-related considerations that most profoundly affects our interactions with our clients and their families is professional ethics. It imposes both restrictions and obligations on our interactions with them. For most professions, these restrictions and obligations are organized into a code of professional ethics to which all persons in the profession are required to adhere. Not doing so can result in a loss of the credential required to practice the profession.

The restrictions and obligations imposed on a practitioner by a code of professional ethics come from several sources. The main one is laws of the community in which the profession is practiced. For ASHA members working in the United States, these would include their municipal, state, and federal laws. They would also include a body of law based on court decisions known as *common law*. The interrelationship between ethics and law is explored in the next section.

INTERRELATIONSHIP BETWEEN ETHICS AND LAW

Law and ethics are interrelated—there is no sharp boundary between them. Ethics (or morality) influences law, which in turn influences how we perceive behavior from an ethical perspective. Consequently, ethics is not an entity that is separate from law but one of the forces that has and will continue to shape laws at all levels in our legal system.

Individuals in our society (as in all others) are encouraged to behave ethically (morally) in their interactions with others. We usually try to avoid interacting with persons whom we believe are not behaving in this manner. This is particularly true for persons from whom we purchase goods and services.

What do we mean when we say that someone's behavior is unethical or immoral? First, we may mean that some aspects of the person's behavior do not conform to our internal standard for what constitutes moral or ethical behavior. Here we are not *describing* behavior. We are making *value judgments* about it. We are saying that it is not what we regard as fair, right, or good. Unfortunately, not everyone agrees on what is fair, right, or good. Consequently, the same act can be viewed as ethical by one person and as unethical by another. Also, a person's internal standard for what is fair, right, or good may not remain constant over time. Furthermore, a person's internal standard for what is fair, right, or good may vary on a *situational basis*. Thus, a person may view a given act as ethical in one situation and as unethical in another.

Second, when we state that someone's behavior is unethical or immoral, we may mean that it is *reputed* to be unethical or immoral. Here we are accepting someone else's value judgment. We are implicitly assuming that another's internal standard for what is fair, right, or good is the same as ours, which may or may not be true. The situation in some instances is even more uncertain because the judgment being communicated is based not on the experience of the person communicating it but on that of someone else. The person is merely reporting what he or she was told.

The *natural law* tradition is the primary avenue through which ethics influence Western legal thought. Although philosophers are not in full agreement about what constitutes natural law, there are some common elements in the ways that they view it. According to Brody,

> what they have in common is the belief in a body of laws governing all people at all times and in a source for those laws other than the customs and institutions of a given society. Such beliefs are frequently accompanied by the additional beliefs that *no societies are authorized to create laws that conflict directly with natural laws, and that such conflicting laws may therefore be invalid* [italics mine]. In

short, the natural law tradition asserts the existence of a set of laws whose status as laws is based on their moral status. (Brody, 1978, pp. 817–818)

Consequently, we use our concept of what is ethical, or moral, both as a standard for assessing the fairness of existing laws and as a guide when encouraging legislators through lobbying (see Chapter 6) to enact new laws. If the majority of the voters in a political unit (a municipality, state, or country) regard an existing law as unfair, they may be able to have it removed by a legislative act. Or if a vocal minority of the voters in a political unit regard an existing situation as unfair, they may be able to convince the members of the appropriate legislature of this unfairness, which may motivate them to pass a law that would at least partially rectify the situation. Parents' groups have used this mechanism to motivate legislatures to pass laws that provide appropriate special education, including speech-language pathology and audiology services, for handicapped children. And advocates for the deaf and severely speech impaired have used it to motivate legislatures to pass laws that provide them with "functionally equivalent" access to telephone communication by mandating and funding telecommunication relay services (Silverman, 1998b).

Thus far in this discussion, ethics has been viewed as a *shaper of law*. The relationship between ethics and law can also be viewed in another way. From this second perspective it can be argued that *ethics is law*—in fact, the *highest* level of law. And consequently, laws enacted by government should not be obeyed if obeying them would result in acts that are immoral—that is, contrary to natural law. You can, in fact, be punished by a court for obeying them. This actually occurred at the Nuremberg trials following World War II. A number of persons in postwar Germany were tried for genocide and convicted. It was argued at these trials that the laws that made the Holocaust possible violated natural law and, consequently, should not have been obeyed. Of course, refusing to obey a law because it violates one's sense of fairness may not be accepted by a court as adequate justification for doing so.

ETHICS AND THE CLINICIAN

Ethical considerations impose restrictions and obligations on both the *delivery of clinical services* and *clinical research*. They come from two sources.

The first is the body of ethical values we all begin to learn as children that govern all aspects of our functioning. Many of them are associated with our religious tradition. And the second is a *code* (or *codes*) *of professional ethics* that we agree to accept when we are certified or licensed. Our failure to abide by it (or them) could result in loss of certification or licensure (see Miller, 1983; Miller & Lubinski, 1986, for information concerning the types of unethical practices that have resulted in such a loss for speech-language pathologists and audiologists).

We will consider in this section the roles that ethical considerations have played historically in regulating clinical functioning. Ethical considerations have been of concern to clinicians for at least the past two thousand years (Konold, 1978). Until the nineteenth century almost all clinicians were physicians, and they regarded the prevention and treatment of communicative disorders to be a part of their clinical responsibility. (Some physicians, particularly those living in Europe who have had a residency in otolaryngology with a sub-specialty in *phoniatrics* still view this as a part of their clinical responsibility.) Since the codes of ethics of almost all nonmedical clinical professions (including speech-language pathology and audiology) were based to some extent on codes of medical ethics, much can be learned about ethical aspects of clinical practice by studying the rationales for certain restrictions on the functioning of a physician that are imposed by medical ethical codes and their precursors—oaths and prayers.

Oaths and Prayers

Many of the restrictions and obligations mentioned in medical ethical codes have their origins in ancient prayers and oaths, particularly the latter. The *Daily Prayer of a Physician*, for example, which is one of the better known of the older statements on medical ethics, includes the following:

> *Do not allow thirst for profit, ambition for renown and admiration, to interfere with my profession, for these are the enemies of truth and of love for mankind and they can lead astray in the great task of attending to the welfare of Thy creatures.*
>
> *Preserve the strength of my body and of my soul that they ever be ready to cheerfully help and support rich and poor, good and bad, enemy as well as friend. In the sufferer let me see only the human being. Illumine my mind that it recognize what presents itself and it may compre-*

hend what is absent or hidden. . . . Let me never be absent-minded. May
no strange thoughts divert my attention at the bedside of the sick, or dis-
turb my mind in its silent labors, for great and sacred are the thought-
ful deliberations required to preserve the . . . health of Thy creatures.
(Friedenwald, 1917, pp. 260–261)

The notion that a clinician needs to "hold paramount the welfare of persons served professionally," which is incorporated into all health care
profession ethical codes in some form is acknowledged in this prayer. The
ethical content of this excerpt, incidentally, would appear to be as relevant
for speech-language pathologists and audiologists as it is for physicians.

Several of the restrictions and obligations that are mentioned in medical ethical codes also are alluded to in medical oaths. The following excerpt from the *Oath of Hippocrates*, which is thought to have been
formulated more than two thousand years ago, is representative.

I will apply dietitic measures for the benefit of the sick according to my
ability and judgment; I will keep them from harm and injustice.

I will neither give a deadly drug to anybody if asked for it nor will I
make a suggestion to this effect. Similarly I will not give a woman an
abortive remedy. In purity and holiness I will guard my life and my art.

I will not use the knife, not even on sufferers from stone, but will
withdraw in favor of such men as are engaged in this work.

Whatever house I may visit, I will come for the benefit of the sick, re-
maining free of all intentional injustices, of all mischief and in particular
of sexual relations with both female and male persons, be they free or slave.

What I may see or hear in the course of the treatment or even out-
side of the treatment in regard to the life of men, which on no account one
must spread abroad, I will keep to myself holding such things shameful
to be spoken about. (Edelstein, 1943, p. 3)

The five paragraphs in this excerpt allude to the ethical principle of "holding paramount the welfare of persons served professionally." A pledge is
made in the first to use one's clinical skills in a manner likely to benefit
one's patients in socially acceptable ways. In the second a pledge is made
not to use one's skills to change a patient in socially unacceptable ways,
even if asked to do so by the patient. Abortion apparently was socially unacceptable when this oath was formulated. During the twentieth century,
it has been socially acceptable at times under certain circumstances. For

this reason, contemporary codes of medical ethics do not forbid physicians to perform abortions under all circumstances. This illustrates an important aspect of professional ethics: What is ethical is not absolute or unchangeable. An act that is viewed as unethical at one point in time may be viewed as ethical at another and vice versa.

A pledge is made in the third paragraph of the oath to make referrals to other professionals when doing so is necessary to provide a patient with the best service possible. One implication of this pledge is that one should not attempt to provide services for which one has been inadequately trained or for which one is not licensed or certified. Physicians were not trained to be surgeons when the *Hippocratic Oath* was formulated: The practice of surgery was a separate profession. Since all of today's physicians are trained to do some surgery, this ethical prohibition is no longer enforced. This further illustrates the point that ethical precepts are not absolute and unchangeable.

A pledge is made in the fourth paragraph of the oath to refrain from intentionally doing anything while functioning clinically that will be detrimental to the patient, regardless of his or her status (e.g., socioeconomic). This prohibition has relevance for doing clinical research on poor people without their knowledge or consent as was done in the syphilis study that was conducted in the United States during the middle of this century in which a number of poor people who had the disease were not treated so that more could be learned about the types of damage syphilis produces (Jones, 1981). And in the fifth, a pledge is made to not reveal what one has learned about a patient or his or her family to unauthorized persons. This precept—that is, confidentiality—is present in some form in all health care profession ethical codes.

Codes of Ethics

While oaths and prayers are likely to affect the ethical behavior of persons who keep them "in mind," they are difficult to enforce. The restrictions and obligations that they place on the activities of practitioners are not usually described specifically enough for violations to be established beyond reasonable doubt. Practitioners may be able to claim with some justification that they didn't realize that what they did was unethical. For this reason and several others, the format currently used in medicine and other health care professions for presenting ethical precepts is a *code of professional ethics*.

The broad ethical concerns addressed in the codes of ethics of most health care professions tend to be quite similar. The results of a survey conducted under the auspices of Georgetown University's Kennedy Institute and the *Encyclopedia of Bioethics* Project of 525 organizations representing a cross section of the health-care professions suggests that the typical code exhorts practitioners

> . . . *to preserve human life, to be a good citizen, to prevent the exploitation of patients, to promote the highest quality health care available, to perform their duties with objectivity and accuracy, to strive for professional excellence through continuing education, to avoid discriminatory practices, to promote the interest and ideals of the profession, to expose unethical and incompetent colleagues, to encourage public health through health-care education, to render service at times of public emergencies, to promote harmonious relations with other health-care professions, and to protect the welfare, dignity, and confidentiality of patients.* (Gass, 1978, p. 1725)

The typical code also provides practitioners with ethical guidelines that address such practical issues relevant to clinical functioning as " . . . advertising, billing procedures, self-aggrandizement [i.e., making oneself appear more knowledgeable and competent than one is], conflicts of interest, professional courtesy, public and media relations, employment and supervision of auxiliary personnel, use of secret remedies and exclusive methods, as well as the location and physical appearance of the office practice" (Gass, 1978, pp. 1725–1726).

It should be apparent from this brief overview that the typical health-care professional code of ethics contains guidelines and precepts that address most aspects of clinical practice. The remainder of this section is devoted to an examination of several of these that are particularly relevant to clinical functioning in speech-language pathology and audiology. The order in which they are discussed does not necessarily reflect their importance.

Confidentiality

One of the most fundamental of all the ethical precepts is the need for confidentiality in the relationship between client and clinician. This need was recognized early in medical ethical thinking as evidenced by its inclusion in the *Oath of Hippocrates*. Originally, this requirement was absolute. Anything that a patient told a physician was supposed to be regarded as confidential and not to be revealed to anyone without the patient's permission. In fact, if a patient told a physician that he or she was going to murder someone, it would have been regarded as unethical for the physician to inform the authorities. Judging by contemporary medical ethical codes (a representative sample of which are included in the appendix of the *Encyclopedia of Bioethics*), this requirement is no longer regarded as absolute. Information obtained from a patient can be revealed without permission under certain circumstances. The American Medical Association's Principles of Medical Ethics, for example, specified three circumstances under which it would not be regarded as unethical to reveal information obtained from a patient without first securing the patient's permission. These are he or she being required to do so by law or because it is necessary to do so to protect the welfare of the individual or the community. These same three exceptions, incidentally, are in the current version of the Code of Ethics of the American Speech-Language-Hearing Association.

The first of these exceptions—being required *by law* to reveal information without the patient's permission—is the one that speech-language pathologists and audiologists are likely to encounter most frequently. Either a civil or criminal court can order them to reveal such information. The likelihood that they could successfully refuse to reveal information requested by a court because they view it as *privileged communication* would depend on the precedents that govern the decisions of the court issuing the order. If a court previously had allowed similar information obtained under similar circumstances to be regarded as privileged communication, it may be willing to do so again. You should consult an attorney to determine the likelihood that a court will honor your refusal to reveal certain information because you regard it as privileged communication.

The second of these exceptions—to protect the welfare of the individual—is apt to be a difficult one to justify. In fact, a clinician would have to assume the *burden of proof* to justify revealing information about a patient without the patient's permission because he or she thought that doing so would protect the patient's welfare. Revealing such information could result in a clinician's being sued by the patient as well as being charged with violating professional ethics. A speech-language pathologist or audiologist would be faced with this type of ethical dilemma when deciding whether to reveal information acquired from a child client to the child's parents. Aside from the possible legal and ethical consequences of revealing information about a client without permission, doing so is unlikely to enhance your relationship with him or her.

The third of these exceptions—to protect the welfare of the community—is apt to be extremely difficult to justify. About the only circumstance under which it would be relatively simple for a clinician to do so would be if a client revealed that he or she was planning to commit a crime. A clinician might with some justification feel an obligation to the community to inform the appropriate authorities.

The confidentiality precept applies to both oral and written communication between client and clinician and includes reports and other clinical records. Information in a client's clinic folder and/or in his or her computer database file(s) should be regarded as confidential, and it ordinarily would be regarded as unethical to release it without his or her permission.

Improvement of Clinical Knowledge and Skills

One precept mentioned in all health-care professional codes of ethics is "holding paramount the welfare of persons served professionally." This implies that the clinician will use the most effective therapy approaches (intervention strategies) available. The American Medical Association in its Principles of Medical Ethics states that "Physicians should strive continually to improve medical knowledge and skill, and should make available to their patients and colleagues the benefits of their professional attainments." This precept, by implication, places several obligations on a clinician. First is an obligation to keep up to date by reading professional journals, attending workshops and conventions, and taking courses (including continuing education courses). The more up-to-date clinicians are in clinical knowledge, the more helpful they are likely to be to their clients. Consequently, failing to keep up to date would be a serious violation of professional ethics because it is incompatible with holding paramount the welfare of one's clients (Carney, 1991).

A second obligation that this precept imposes on a clinician is to evaluate the effectiveness of his or her intervention strategies. Doing so would tend to increase a clinician's effectiveness (assuming, of course, that intervention strategies that were not effective would be modified or discarded). For a discussion of this and other reasons why it is desirable for clinicians to systematically assess and document therapy outcome, see Chapter 2 in Silverman (1998a).

A third obligation that this ethical precept imposes on a clinician is to advance clinical knowledge and techniques if he or she has an opportunity to do so. One way that a clinician can do this is by sharing information with other clinicians about the impacts (both positive and negative) that some of the therapy programs and techniques he or she has used have had on clients (while, of course, not violating the legal/ethical requirements for confidentiality). A case for why it is necessary for clinicians to share such information if they are to "hold paramount the welfare of persons served professionally" is outlined in Silverman (1998a).

Truth-Telling and Informed Consent

A clinician has an obligation to be honest with patients about the nature of their condition, the prognosis for improvement, and the possible impacts (both positive and negative) of therapy. A clinician may have a similar obligation to the families of patients, particularly when patients are children or severely impaired adults who are unable to understand the information or to whom receipt of such information is likely to be detrimental. The ethical ramifications of telling the truth have been dealt with extensively in the medical literature, particularly with regard to the desirability of informing a patient that he or she is dying. The arguments for and against truth-telling are summarized below.

One of the main arguments in favor of truth-telling is that a patient has the right to decide whether he or she wishes to participate in the intervention program recommended by a clinician. Unless the patient has been given accurate information about the nature of his or her condition, its prognosis, and the probable impacts (both positive and negative) of the intervention program (or alternative intervention programs), the patient's consent to participate in the program is unlikely to be viewed by a court as being legally binding. On the other hand, if a patient is given such information, a court is likely to view his or her consent to participate as being *informed consent* and consequently, legally binding. The assumption, of course, is being made here that the person can understand the information being presented—that is, he or she does not have a neurological condition (such as receptive aphasia, mental retardation, Alzheimer's disease, cerebral arteriosclerosis) or a hearing loss and understands English well. It is also being assumed that he or she is not a young child.

One of the main arguments against truth-telling, especially complete truth-telling, is that it can have a detrimental effect on the patient. If a patient is told the prognosis for improvement is poor, the therapy may be less beneficial than it would have been if he or she had been given a less truthful or less complete statement of prognosis. That is, he or she may reject therapy or become so despondent that he or she cannot benefit maximally from it.

This situation illustrates a type of ethical dilemma in which there are two possible courses of action, either of which can result in our violating an ethical principle. If a patient is given an honest statement of prognosis, it may have a detrimental effect, thus violating the ethical principle that the welfare of persons served professionally must be paramount. On the other hand, if a patient is not given a completely truthful statement of prognosis because such a statement would be likely to have a detrimental effect, this would violate the ethical principle that a clinician should be truthful with patients. A clinician who is confronted by such a situation would have to weigh the competing ethical considerations to determine the violation of which would be likely to be least detrimental to the patient.

One aspect of truth-telling that is mentioned in a number of health-care professional codes of ethics is not guaranteeing cures. Many variables can influence how much a patient will improve, and a clinician can rarely predict their impacts with accuracy.

Informed consent is also an important ethical consideration for *clinical research*. Persons must be fully informed about potential risks when they are asked to participate in a research project. Not doing so can result in both your being sued and criminal prosecution.

Not Exploiting Persons Served Professionally

All health-care professional codes of ethics implicitly or explicitly prohibit practitioners from exploiting those whom they are serving professionally. Such exploitation can arise from several sources. One is the fees charged for services rendered. The American Medical Associations's Principles of Medical Ethics, for example, includes the following statement:

> *In the practice of medicine a physician should limit the source of his professional income to medical services actually rendered by him, or under his supervision, to his patients. His fee should be commensurate with the services rendered and the patient's ability to pay. He should neither pay or receive a commission for referral of patients. Drugs, remedies, or appliances may be dispensed or supplied by the physician provided it is in the best interests of the patient.*

Consequently, a practitioner would be exploiting those whom he or she is serving professionally by charging fees that are higher than would be commensurate with the services he or she rendered and the client's ability to pay. He or she would also be exploiting them by paying or receiving a commission for referring clients to other practitioners, by selling them things they do not need, or for charging them for services not rendered.

The fee for a health-care service may be paid by a third party—an insurance agency—rather than the patient. This ethical prohibition still applies. This is, it is unethical to charge an insurance agency a fee for services not rendered or a higher fee than is commensurate with the services rendered.

A second source of such exploitation is accepting patients for treatment or continuing treatment when the prognosis for improvement (or further improvement) is extremely poor. Private practitioners and those employed by for-profit agencies are particularly likely to be tempted to do this if their caseloads are relatively small and discharging or refusing patients will result in a loss of income. It makes no difference whether the fees charged for treating them are being billed to a third party (an insurance program) or to the patients themselves. Remember, the persons who ultimately pay for excess fees billed to insurance programs are you and the other members of general public.

Monitoring Compliance with the Code of Ethics
Health-care professional codes of ethics require practitioners to report violations to the board that monitors compliance with it. The following statement from the American Medical Association's Principles of Medical Ethics is representative:

> *The medical profession should safeguard the public and itself against physicians deficient in moral character or professional competence. Physicians should observe all laws, uphold the dignity and honor of the profession and its self-imposed disciplines. They should expose, without hesitation, illegal or unethical conduct of fellow members of the profession.*

This obligation is a logical consequence of accepting what is probably the most fundamental of all these ethical requirements—holding paramount the welfare of persons served professionally. The persons whose welfare you are obliged to hold paramount are not just the ones in your caseload (Koenigsknecht, 1990a). For speech-language pathologists and audiologists, they would include all persons who are communicatively impaired (see Koenigsknecht, 1990b; National forum on consumer rights, 1990). Consequently, holding paramount the welfare of persons served professionally obliges you to expose the unethical conduct and incompetence of fellow professionals. Of course, if you charge a fellow professional with being unethical or incompetent, you must either be prepared to prove it or to provide sufficient evidence to justify an investigation. Otherwise, you may find yourself the defendant in a defamation suit.

Patient Selection and Discrimination

To what extent is it permissible for clinicians to choose whom they will and will not serve? Is it always unethical to consider race, cultural background, religion, sex, and ability to pay? Is it unethical to exclude from ones caseload persons who have a particular disease, such as AIDS? These questions are answered somewhat differently in the various health-care professional codes of ethics. In some, such as the American Medical Association's Principles of Ethics, they are dealt with directly and the clinician is allowed considerable freedom in patient selection:

> *A physician may choose whom he will serve. In an emergency, however, he should render service to the best of his ability.*

In others, such as the American Psychological Association's Ethical Standards for Psychologists (Reich, 1978, pp. 1811–1815), they are dealt with indirectly, if at all. And in still others, such as the Code of Ethics of the American Speech-Language-Hearing Association , they are dealt with directly and clinicians are prohibited from discriminating against clients on certain bases:

> *Individuals must not discriminate in the delivery of professional services on any basis that is unjustifiable or irrelevant to the need for and potential benefit from such services, such as race, sex, age, religion, national origin, sexual orientation, or handicapping condition.*

There is one area of possible discrimination that does not currently appear to be addressed directly in many health-care professional codes of ethics. This is choosing not to provide services (or to provide only limited services) to persons whose bills are paid by some third parties, such as governmental insurance programs (e.g., Medicare and Medicaid). The fees they pay for certain services are sometimes considerably lower than those usually charged for them, and providing services to those covered by such programs tends to entail a relatively large amount of paperwork. Also, the agencies responsible for administering these programs may be relatively slow in paying, which can cause cash-flow problems. This issue is addressed indirectly in some health-care professional codes of ethics: The American Medical Association in its Principles of Medical Ethics, for example, states that fees charged "should be commensurate with . . . the patient's ability to pay." This statement would appear to imply that a patient should not be denied services because the fees that the patient can be charged are lower than the practitioner's usual ones. The ethical issues here are murky, and clinicians will have to rely on their own sense of what is fair or on the fee policies of their employers when deciding whether to serve such patients.

Advertising

Most health-care professional codes of ethics place some restrictions on the advertising of clinical services, but not as many as previously. The first Code of Ethics of the American Medical Association (1847), which served as the model for subsequent health-care professional codes of ethics in the United States, placed the following restrictions on the advertising of such services:

> It is derogatory to the dignity of the profession, to resort to public advertisement or private cards or handbills, inviting the attention of individuals affected with particular diseases— publicly offering advice and medicine to the poor gratis, or promising radical cures; to publish cases and operations in the daily prints, or suffer such publications to be made;—to invite laymen to be present at operations—to boast of cures and remedies—to adduce certificates of skill and success, or to perform any similar acts. These are the ordinary practices of empirics [charlatans and quacks], and are highly reprehensible to a regular physician. (Reich, 1978, pp. 1741–1742)

It would appear from this excerpt that the original impetus for restricting advertising was to differentiate the trained practitioner from the charlatan or quack (Ciuccio, 1990). (The term *quack*, as used here, refers to a practitioner who lacks the qualifications and training regarded as necessary by proponents of the profession's licensure and certification requirements. There have been at least a few cases in which a practitioner who was viewed as a *quack* was later viewed as an *innovator*.)

Restrictions on the advertising of clinical services have been relaxed somewhat during the past twenty years (Ciuccio, 1990). There appear to be several reasons why these restrictions were relaxed. First, there is an obvious need to make people aware of who is a qualified practitioner. If only unqualified practitioners are permitted to advertise their services, the public will have difficulty locating qualified ones. Thus, physicians and other health-care professionals (including speech-language pathologists and audiologists) were permitted to list themselves under appropriate headings in the *Yellow Pages* of the telephone book and to discreetly inform both the public and professionals in the community who may serve as referral sources about their services. In some health-care fields (e.g., medicine) restrictions on advertising have been relaxed to the point where it is no longer regarded as unethical for practitioners to advertise their services on television.

A second reason for relaxing restrictions on advertising is that such restrictions have been viewed by the courts as constituting *restraint of trade* (Ciuccio, 1990). From this perspective, restrictions on advertising keep costs to consumers high by eliminating competition among practitioners. If practitioners were to directly or indirectly advertise the costs of their services, consumers probably would consider cost when selecting a practitioner. Consequently, practitioners would have some motivation to keep their fees reasonable, which, at least theoretically, would tend to lower costs to consumers. Since the advertising of fees for professional services is a relatively recent phenomenon, it is uncertain how much impact it actually will have on the costs of such services.

CODE OF ETHICS OF THE AMERICAN SPEECH-LANGUAGE-HEARING ASSOCIATION

The Code of Ethics of the American Speech-Language-Hearing Association (ASHA) has much in common with those of other health-care professions. It imposes on speech-language pathologists and audiologists all of the restrictions and obligations that have been discussed here. And like the others, it has evolved considerably since its initial formulation.

Ethical issues have been of concern to ASHA since the founding of the Association in 1925. In fact, one of the reasons mentioned for founding the organization, according to Paden, was "To establish scientific standards and *codes of ethics* [italics mine]" (1970, p. 73). The relatively high level of concern that the founders of ASHA had about professional ethics was, at least in part, a reaction to the unprofessional conduct of some practitioners who treated speech disorders, especially stuttering.

> *Such persons were known, for example, to make rash guarantees of cure, to require their patients to sign statements that they would never reveal their methods, to charge exorbitant fees, and to otherwise degrade the image of the profession.* (Paden, 1970, p. 73)

Also, a few were known to treat speech disorders completely or almost completely by correspondence. Many of the practices that were prohibited in the various revisions of the ASHA ethical code were a part of the modus operandi of some nineteenth- and early twentieth-century practitioners.

The primary ethical focus during the early years of ASHA seemed to have been on preventing unethical practitioners from joining rather than on monitoring the ethical practices of members. This may partially explain why, prior to 1950, statements about ethics were included in the section of the Association's constitution that dealt with membership requirements rather than in a separate document. This focus also is evident from the qualifications for membership that were included in the original (1926) constitution of the Association. There were five qualifications listed, one of which was the following:

> *Possession of a professional reputation untainted by a past record (or a present record) of unethical practices such as blatant commercialization of professional services, or guaranteeing of "cures" for stated sums of money.*

It apparently was not until the early 1940s that the Association was called upon to investigate a complaint about the ethical practices of a member (Paden, 1970). (For further information about the early development of the ASHA Code of Ethics, see Paden, 1970.)

The primary ethical focus of ASHA at the present time (as it seems to have been since the 1950s) is on monitoring the ethical practices of its members. All members who are engaged in clinical practice and all non-members who have ASHA clinical certification are required to agree to be bound by the Code of Ethics. The change in focus from admission to membership to monitoring of membership appears to have come about largely because most persons who joined ASHA after the 1940s had not had sufficient paid clinical experience for their ethical standards to be assessed. Most of those who sought membership during the early years had been functioning as practitioners for a significant period of time, which made it possible to assess their ethical standards prior to admitting them to membership.

The issues addressed in the various revisions of the ASHA Code parallel those addressed in other health-care professional codes of ethics at the same points in time. This has occurred because the health-care professions have had to cope with similar ethical problems during given time periods. During the 1970s, for example, a number of these professions had to cope with ethical problems associated with their practitioners' treating patients whose therapy is paid for by a *third party*, such as Medicare or Medicaid. Most of the issues that are addressed in the ASHA Code are discussed elsewhere in this chapter.

Codes of ethics deal with *general principles of ethical behavior*. The application of these general principles to specific situations encountered by clinicians often requires some interpretation. A series of articles has appeared in ASHA publications over the years (mostly in the journal *Asha*), some with titles beginning *Issues in Ethics*, that have attempted to interpret how the ASHA Code can be applied to certain situations encountered by clinicians, including the following: *third-party payment* (Bangs, 1970); *advertising of members' products* (Issues in ethics: Advertising of members' products, 1974); *honoring of contracts* (Issues in ethical practice—Responsibilities concerning the honoring of a verbal or written contract, 1958); *fees for clinical services provided by students* (Issues in ethics: Fees for clinical services provided by students, 1978); *action by ASHA for violation of state association or licensure ethical codes* (Issues in ethics—Ethical practice inquiries: State versus ASHA decision differences, 1978); *speech-language pathologists functioning as audiologists and vice versa* (Issues in ethics: Clinical practice by certificate holders in areas in which they are not certified, 1986); *CFY supervisors' responsibilities* (Issues in ethics: CFY supervisors' responsibilities, 1980a); *degrees from "diploma mills"* (Issues in ethics: The bogus degree, 1974); *use of supportive personnel* (Issues in ethics: ASHA policy re: supportive personnel, 1979); *public statements and announcements by members* (Issues in ethics: Public announcements and public statements, 1981); *ASHA members who are uncertified engaging in clinical practice* (Issues in ethics: Identification of members engaged in clinical practice without certification, 1973), *listing in telephone directories* (Issues in ethics: Guidelines for telephone directories, 1974); *gratuities* (Issues in ethics: Gratuities, 1978); *private practice* (Issues in ethics: Drawing cases for private practice from primary place of employment, 1980b); *research* (Issues in ethics: Ethics in research and professional practice, 1982); *use of graduate degrees* (Issues in ethics: Use of graduate degrees by members and/or certificate holders, 1987); *competition* (Issues in ethics: Competition, 1989a); *prescription* (Issues in ethics: Prescription, 1989b); and *supervision of student clinicians* (Issues in ethics: Supervision of student clinicians, 1991).

While the ASHA Code of Ethics provides guidelines for dealing with most situations a speech-language pathologist or audiologist is likely to encounter, all situations are not covered. For example, consider the following scenario: A speech-language pathologist after being hired to supervise a public school system clinical service program discovers that there are two or three staff members at the BA level offering direct services. The state views these persons as qualified, but ASHA doesn't agree. How should he or she handle the situation?

The *Ethical Practice Board* (EPB) is responsible for investigating charges of code violations by ASHA members (see Ethical Practice Board statement of practices and procedures, 1991). If the preponderance of evidence following a careful investigation suggests that the member did violate the Code of Ethics, the board can recommend that disciplinary action of some kind be taken. The most extreme action that it can recommend is revocation of membership and certification (see *Actions of the Ethical Practice Board*, 1986, 1988, 1989a, 1989b, 1991a, 1991b, 1991c). Information about procedures for filing or answering a complaint can be obtained from the ASHA national office. Anyone who has been accused of violating the ASHA Code and is being investigated by EPB would probably be wise to consult with an attorney.

REFERENCES

Actions of the Ethical Practice Board. (1986). *Asha*, 28 (7), 51.
Actions of the Ethical Practice Board. (1988). *Asha*, 30 (1), 59.
Actions of the Ethical Practice Board. (1989a). *Asha*, 31 (9), 47.
Actions of the Ethical Practice Board. (1989b). *Asha*, 31 (11), 59.
Actions of the Ethical Practice Board. (1991a). *Asha*, 33 (1), 68.
Actions of the Ethical Practice Board. (1991b). *Asha*, 33 (4), 70.

Actions of the Ethical Practice Board. (1991c). *Asha,* 33 (8), 55.

Bangs, J. L. (1970). Third party payment abuses. *Asha,* 12, 418.

Brody, B. A. (1978). Law and morality. In W. T. Reich (Ed.), *Encyclopedia of Bioethics,* Volume 2. New York: Free Press.

Carney, P. J. (1991). Competence: An ethical decision. *Asha,* 33 (4), 7–8.

Ciuccio, J. (1990). Ethics, nostrums, and quackery. *Asha,* 33 (8), 38–39.

Edelstein, L. (1943). The Hippocratic Oath: Text, translation, and interpretation. *Bulletin of the History of Medicine,* Supplement 1. Baltimore, MD: Johns Hopkins University Press.

Ethical Practice Board statement of practices and procedures. (1991). *Asha,* 33 (3), 105–106.

Friedenwald, H. (1917). *Bulletin of the Johns Hopkins Hospital,* 28, 260–261.

Gass, R. S. (1978). Codes of the health-care professions. In W. T. Reich (Ed.), *Encyclopedia of Bioethics,* Volume 4. New York: Free Press.

Issues in ethical practice—responsibilities concerning the honoring of a verbal or written contract. (1958). *Journal of Speech and Hearing Disorders,* 23, 160–161.

Issues in ethics: Identification of members engaged in clinical practice without certification. (1973). *Asha,* 15, 381.

Issues in ethics: Advertising of members' products. (1974). *Asha,* 16, 44.

Issues in ethics: The bogus degree. (1974). *Asha,* 16, 212.

Issues in ethics: CFY supervisors' responsibilities (1974). *Asha,* 16, 212.

Issues in ethics: Guidelines for telephone directories. (1974). *Asha,* 16, 708–709.

Issues in ethics: Gratuities. (1978). *Asha,* 20, 311–312.

Issues in ethics: Fees for clinical services provided by students. (1978). *Asha,* 20, 427.

Issues in ethics: Ethical practice inquiries: State versus ASHA decision differences. (1978). *Asha,* 20, 505–506.

Issues in ethics: ASHA policy re. supportive personnel. (1979). *Asha,* 21, 419.

Issues in ethics: CFY supervisors' responsibilities. (1980a). *Asha,* 22, 273–274.

Issues in ethics: Drawing cases for private practice from primary place of employment. (1980b). *Asha,* 22, 939.

Issues in ethics: Public announcements and public statements. (1981). *Asha,* 23, 107.

Issues in ethics: Ethics in research and professional practice. (1982). *Asha,* 24, 1029–1031.

Issues in ethics: Clinical practice by certificate holders in areas in which they are not certified. (1986). *Asha,* 28 (4), 58.

Issues in ethics: Use of graduate degrees by members and/or certificate holders. (1987). *Asha,* 29 (6), 42.

Issues in ethics: Competition. (1989a). *Asha,* 31 (9), 45.

Issues in ethics: Prescription. (1989b). *Asha,* 31 (9), 45.

Issues in ethics: Supervision of student clinicians. (1991). *Asha,* 33 (10), 53.

Jones, J. H. (1981). *Bad Blood: The Tuskegee Syphilis Experiment.* New York: The Free Press.

Koenigsknecht, R. A. (1990a). Ethics: For goodness sake. *Asha*, 32 (9), 7–8.

Koenigsknecht, R. A. (1990b). Learn from our consumers. *Asha*, 32 (6), 33–34.

Konold, D. (1978). Codes of medical ethics: I. History. In W. T. Reich (Ed.), *Encyclopedia of Bioethics*, Volume 1. New York: Free Press.

Miller, T. D. (1983). *Professional Liability in Speech-Language Pathology and Audiology: Unprofessional Conduct and Unethical Practice*. Unpublished doctoral dissertation, State University of New York at Buffalo.

Miller, T. D., & Lubinski, R. (1986). Professional liability in speech-language pathology and audiology. *Asha*, 28 (6), 45–47.

National forum on consumer rights. (1990). *Asha*, 32 (6), 35–39.

Paden, E. P. (1970). *A History of the American Speech and Hearing Association, 1925–1958*. Rockville, MD: American Speech-Language-Hearing Association.

Reich, W. T. (Ed.) (1978). *Encyclopedia of Bioethics, Volume 4*. New York: Free Press.

Silverman, F. H. (1998a). *Research Design and Evaluation in Speech-Language Pathology and Audiology* (4th ed.). Boston: Allyn & Bacon.

Silverman, F. H. (1998b). *The Telecommunication Relay Service (TRS) Handbook*. Newport, RI: Aegis Publishing Group.

▶ 3

Credentialing—Licensure, Certification, Registration, and Accreditation

One of the ways that society influences the clinical functioning of speech-language pathologists and audiologists is through the mechanisms of licensure, certification, registration, and accreditation. These define both the populations to whom speech-language pathologists and audiologists can offer services and the types of services that they can offer them. A person credentialed as an audiologist would be permitted to provide certain services to certain populations (e.g., fitting hearing aids to persons who have hearing losses) that a person credentialed as a speech-language pathologist would ordinarily not be permitted to provide and vice versa. Licensure, certification, and registration also place restrictions on *how services are provided* by requiring adherence to a code of ethics. Failure to function in a manner consistent with such a code can result in your credential being taken away (e.g., Actions of the Ethical Practices Board, 1986, 1988, 1989a, 1989b, 1991). In addition, licensure, certification, and registration impose restrictions on how practitioners are *trained*. The requirements for the Certificates of Clinical Competence in Speech-Language Pathology and Audiology awarded by the American Speech-Language-Hearing Association and state licensure and registration (including that needed to work in the public schools) influence the curriculums of speech-language pathology and audiology training programs. Finally, credentialing requirements can influence how speech-language pathologists and audiologists are *paid for their services*. Some health insurance programs (e.g., Medicare) stipulate that for speech-language pathology services to be covered they must be provided by a practitioner who has met the requirements for ASHA Certification or other appropriate credential. Also, if a school district wants to be reimbursed by the state for services it provides children who are communicatively impaired, the services must be provided by speech-language pathologists who are credentialed by the state department of public instruction.

MOTIVATION FOR INITIATING LICENSURE, CERTIFICATION, REGISTRATION, AND ACCREDITATION

Whenever individuals or groups try to change the status quo, it is almost always because they expect to derive some benefit from doing so. Their expectations may or may not be realistic. The reasons that they give for wanting the change may not be the real ones or all of them. Rather, they may be reasons that they believe will be regarded as compelling by those who must approve the change.

The regulation of professionals through licensure, certification, accreditation, and registration in the United States is a relatively recent phenomenon historically. In the health field it appears to have begun with medicine. Prior to 1800 many states attempted to regulate medical practice with varying degrees of success. It was not until just before the Civil War, however, that interest in regulating health professionals reached a national level with the establishment of the American Medical Association in 1847 and the American Dental Association in 1859 (Levine, 1978). Practitioners in most other health-related fields (including speech-language pathology and audiology) were not regulated prior to the twentieth century.

The individuals and groups who seek regulation for an occupation (particularly a profession) tend to be those who are members of it rather than consumers of its services. The investment required for achieving some form of regulation is usually substantial—with regard to both time and money. Since regulation would be expected to place restrictions on the activities of those seeking it, why would they be motivated to pursue it? What *benefits* would they expect to receive from achieving it? My intent in this section is to provide at least a partial answer to these questions. According to Rottenberg (1968, p. 283):

> *The primary justification that usually is given for regulating an occu-pation is the protection of public health, safety, or morals. Those seeking regulation argue that without it, incompetent practitioners will offer their services. Prospective buyers of these services are said not to be able to distinguish between qualified and unqualified persons, and this is considered to be especially true if consumers buy services of the particu-lar kind only at infrequent intervals. Where the consequences of the em-ployment of unqualified persons can be expected to be seriously aversive to the purchaser, and especially where the consequences of incompetently rendered service are irreversible, it is thought to be desirable that . . . some examining or other procedure [be administered] to determine who are qualified to practice, and prevent those who are unqualified from of-fering their services. The average quality of those permitted to practice is raised, and by exclusion of "quacks" and incompetents the public is protected from the error of employing them.*

While these arguments were initially formulated to promote licensing, they have been used as justification for other forms of regulation as well.

Credentialing can be justified on the basis that it tends to raise the av-erage quality of the services offered by the members of a profession. How-ever, this may not be the only reason or even the main reason why the members of a profession pursue it. Their primary motivation may be to gain *legal status*, or recognition, for their profession:

> *Once a profession is awarded legal status and is given the exclusive right to practice in the field of its competence, it can inhibit the practice of im-postors by taking action in the courts. . . . Each profession defines an area of practice in which it has a monopoly and fights hard to preserve that unique area.* (Lum, 1979, p. 156)

Thus, by gaining legal status through regulation a health profession can establish what its members hope will be an *exclusive* claim to a segment of the health service territory. The total territory consists of all services for preventing and ameliorating all the disorders that a person can develop; each profession is seeking to be granted the exclusive right to provide *cer-*

tain of these services to those who have *certain* disorders. If they are successful, they will have a monopoly (or close to a monopoly) on the delivery of certain services to the segment of the territory to which they have staked a claim. Medicine is an example of a profession that has been successful in establishing a near monopoly on the delivery of certain services to a segment of this territory.

When a profession is awarded a monopoly (or close to a monopoly) for the delivery of certain services, it is expected to see to it that these services are provided in a responsible manner. According to Lum,

> *Society accords a monopoly to a profession with respect to its practice and standard setting on the premise that no lay person understands esoteric knowledge on which the profession rests, and therefore no lay person can judge what should be done. Society allows a profession to hold a monopoly because it is convinced that the profession is dedicated to an ethical or altruistic ideal in serving society. Society continues to allow this monopoly as long as it is convinced that a profession is exercising its privileges responsibly and aids and/or serves its clientele without exploitation.*
>
> *Under its monopoly, a profession has the purpose of protecting not only the society it serves, but also its members, making it possible for them to practice effectively. Its protection, which occurs through methods passed on by socialization, takes different form as the profession confronts internal as well as external dangers.*
>
> *Internally, a profession must protect society and its members against the incompetent or dishonest member whose actions may damage trust in the profession. A profession controls the number and kinds of persons who are allowed to enter and to study through the establishment of admission criteria and determining the length and types of programs allowed. These controls are imposed in order to prevent incompetent persons from entering the profession and to avoid an oversupply of practitioners as well. In addition, it controls the body of knowledge on which the practice rests and maintains the quality and standards of its education through a process of external accreditation. It further controls admission to the profession through licensing procedures as well as through various certification and credential procedures. It opposes efforts to establish conditions that would make its practice difficult or impossible. Each profession has an obligation to police its own ranks*

*and make certain that those who wear the name and display the license
are in fact ethical and competent practitioners. From this obligation stem
efforts to enforce the code of ethics of the profession even to the extent of
expelling members who flagrantly violate provisions of its code. Thus, a
physician can have his [or her] license revoked and a lawyer can be "dis-
barred." Professional associations aid practitioners in obtaining legal
sanction for their monopoly.* (Lum, 1979, pp. 155–156)

In a sense, when a profession is granted a monopoly, it enters into a contract with the community (through the legislature) that granted it. As
compensation for the legal status accorded it, the members of the profession agree to provide certain services that are of an acceptable quality. If
they fail to do what they promised, the community has the right (perhaps
even the obligation) to terminate their monopoly as providers of these services.

One possible consequence of regulating the practice of a profession is
reducing the number of persons entering it. The higher the cost to qualify
as a practitioner, the less likely persons are to attempt to do so if they do
not expect the financial rewards from qualifying to be worth the investment. Several factors are likely to contribute to the cost of entering a profession. The most obvious one is the cost of the training or education
needed to do so. In addition to this expense, there is also an indirect one—
the money the person would have earned if he or she had worked instead.
Furthermore, a substantial time and energy investment is necessary.

When the members of a professional group recommend requirements
for a new credential or new requirements for an existing credential, it is
not uncommon for them to make these requirements *more demanding* than
those they were required to satisfy, and if their recommendations are accepted, to award themselves the new (or revised) license or certificate
through a *grandfather clause*. Such clauses stimulate "that those who have
already entered and are practicing the occupation be qualified *pro forma*
and exempted from examination" (Rottenberg, 1968, p. 283). The term *pro
forma* in this context is used to suggest that the credential is awarded not
on the basis of a conviction that those awarded it under the grandfather
clause are qualified, but merely to facilitate acceptance of it by existing
practitioners. Changes in the requirements for a credential would be unlikely to be acceptable to them if their adoption meant that they would no
longer qualify to be practitioners.

REGULATION OF OCCUPATIONS

Several types of credentials can be used to regulate an occupation. Some are initiated and administered by a professional association and others by a government agency (usually a state one). Each is described in this section.

Types of Credentials Administered by a Professional Organization

A professional association can regulate the practice of an occupation in two main ways: through certification and accreditation. Both are used by the American Speech-Language-Hearing Association to regulate the practice of speech-language pathology and audiology.

Certification

Certification is "a voluntary mechanism by which a nongovernmental agency or association grants recognition to an individual who has met certain predetermined qualifications specified by that agency or association" (Roemer, 1974, p. 26). Because certification is a *voluntary* mechanism, persons who are not certified in an occupation can legally enter it (assuming that no license is required). They may, however, have difficulty finding employment because employers may refuse to hire those who do not have the certification, for several reasons. First, certification simplifies the hiring process. Its possession by an applicant both indicates and documents that his or her education and experience is adequate to meet at least minimum acceptable performance standards. Second, it may make it easier to secure payments from *third parties* (such as private and government-sponsored insurance programs) for clinical services. [This also applies for licensure—see White, 1986.] Some third-party payers may stipulate that they will only pay for services that are provided or supervised by persons who are certified as competent by the national association to which members of the profession belong. (An example of such an association would be the American Speech-Language-Hearing Association).

Certification may be offered by professional associations to document *specialty* qualifications in addition to, or instead of, basic ones. When all states regulate the practice of a profession on a basic level through licensure (as is the case in medicine), then professional organizations tend to concentrate their efforts on *specialty certification*. (A specialty for which certification is offered in medicine is otolaryngology.) Consequently, when all states regulate the practice of speech-language pathology and audiology through licensure, the American Speech-Language-Hearing Association is likely to emphasize specialty certification (e.g., for treating fluency disorders) rather than its present certification program.

Certification can be offered for a *relatively narrow* subject matter specialty, such as administering and interpreting a particular test or using a specific intervention approach. While organizations that award this type of certification cannot legally prevent uncertified persons from using their tests or intervention strategies, they can make it difficult for them to do so by making full sets of materials available only to those who are certified or in the process of becoming certified.

Most professional certification programs have several components in addition to requiring adherence of a code of ethics. First, they require the successful completion of one or more courses that many or may not be offered for academic credit by a college or university. Second, they usually require a specified minimum amount of supervised practical (practicum) experience. Third, they may require an "internship" following completion of the academic and practicum requirements. Fourth, they may require the passing of an examination. And fifth, they may require persons who have the certification to expose themselves periodically to continuing education. (The words *expose themselves* were used because most continuing education courses do not have examinations or other mechanisms for determining how much participants have learned.) The American Speech-Language-Hearing Association's Certificates of Clinical Competence in Speech-Language Pathology and Audiology require the first four of these components. The fifth is encouraged through awarding of the ACE certificate.

While certification encourages practitioners to obtain the training necessary to perform their services competently and to behave ethically in their interactions with others, it has several limitations as a mechanism for insuring competence. According to Roemer,

> *The basic requirement for certification is completion of an approved educational program, but the multiplicity of educational programs in different settings for the same occupation makes surveillance difficult. For many health occupations, no substitution of work experience or recognition of equivalent qualifications is allowed in place of academic quali-*

fications for certification. Very few certifying bodies use examinations developed by professional testing agencies. [ASHA does use such examinations for its certification program.] In some cases, use of proficiency examinations might be a better measure of skills than written examinations. Not all certifying bodies require continuing quality of performance by persons certified, though they may require continuing membership in the association. (1974, p. 29)

Accreditation

A second approach that a professional organization can use for regulating the practice of an occupation is to *establish standards* for the curriculum and administration of programs that train new practitioners. Such programs may be offered by a college or university or by some other institution. (A hospital school of nursing would be an example of a professional training program that is offered by an institution other than a college or university.) By influencing the curriculums of programs that are training the practitioners for a profession, a professional organization can influence both the number of new persons who enter it and how they are trained.

A professional organization can influence the numbers of new practitioners entering a field in several ways. First, it can control the amount of education a person has to obtain before he or she is employable as a practitioner. The greater the amount beyond a certain level (e.g., a bachelor's degree), the fewer the number of persons who probably will be interested in entering the field, particularly if there are other fields offering similar rewards for which entrance is less costly.

A professional organization can also influence the number of new practitioners entering a field by limiting the number and size of training programs. It can, for example, make such programs sufficiently expensive to discourage some universities and colleges from beginning, continuing, or expanding them by requiring low maximum faculty–student ratios.

By controlling curriculum, a professional association can influence how practitioners in accredited programs are trained. It can influence the training of others as well. For example, the curriculum established by the American Speech-Language-Hearing Association influences the training of students who graduate from unaccredited programs and are licensed by a state department of public instruction as speech-language clinicians. It even influences how foreign practitioners are trained (see Silverman & Moulton, 1997).

What is accreditation and how does it function? Accreditation is "the process by which an agency or organization evaluates or recognizes a program of study or an institution as meeting certain predetermined qualifications or standards" (Standards for federal funding, 1972, p. 547). The agency or organization is not directly (or officially) affiliated with any municipal, state, or federal governmental unit. It may, however, be indirectly affiliated with one or more such units. One way that this can occur is by an agency or organization being officially recognized by a governmental unit as the regional or national accrediting body for a specific type of institution (e.g., a college or a hospital) or for a particular program offered by one. (Colleges and universities, incidentally, are evaluated and accredited overall—as a totality—by one of six regional or national accrediting associations, each of which is responsible for colleges and universities located in a particular geographical region of the United States—e.g., the Middle States Association of Colleges and Schools.)

Two groups that can recognize accrediting organizations or agencies as "reliable authorities as to the quality of training offered by educational institutions" (Standards for federal funding, 1972, p. 547) are the Council on Postsecondary Accreditation and the U.S. Commissioner of Education. Both have recognized the American Speech-Language-Hearing Association as "the national accrediting agency for college and university programs offering *master's degrees* [italics mine] in speech pathology and audiology" (Standards for federal funding, 1972, p. 548). There were no organizations or agencies specifically accrediting baccalaurate or doctoral programs in these fields when this chapter was written.

Whether a college or university training program is accredited by an organization recognized by a national governmental unit can affect the flow of federal dollars to that program. Accreditation by such a body has sometimes been made a requirement for eligibility to participate in funding programs sponsored by agencies of the federal government, including those providing training grants. The Social and Rehabilitation Services Program of the Department of Health, Education, and Welfare during the early 1970s, for example, proposed to include the following in its list of criteria for determining eligibility for speech-language pathology and audiology training programs to participate in their training grants program:

> *In order for master's degree programs to be eligible for support, they should be accredited, or be in the process of review for accreditation, by*

the American Speech and Hearing Association [now the American Speech-Language-Hearing Association] through the American Board of Examiners in Speech Pathology and Audiology and its Education and Training Board. (Standards for federal funding, 1972, p. 546)

The use of such a criterion when determining eligibility of training programs for federal support has been questioned on the basis that it tends to create a *Catch-22* situation—that is, some unaccredited programs probably could be strengthened sufficiently with federal support to achieve accreditation, but their lack of accreditation impedes their securing the federal support they need to strengthen their curriculums. Such a situation was claimed to have existed during the early 1970s for some speech-language pathology and audiology training programs in predominantly black institutions (Standards for federal funding, 1972).

The functioning of both institutional and programmatic accrediting organizations is being subjected to increasing scrutiny. Their decisions are more frequently being viewed as judgments make by human beings (in most cases, human beings who are attempting to function in a relatively unbiased manner) rather than as facts or truths.

For additional information about accreditation of speech-language pathology and audiology master's degree training programs, see *Standards for accreditation of educational programs* (1990).

Types of Regulation Administered by a Governmental Agency

There are three main ways by which a governmental agency can regulate the practice of an occupation: individual licensure, institutional licensure, and registration. The first was used most often to regulate the practice of speech-language pathology and audiology when this chapter was written.

Individual Licensure

Individual licensing laws are "a legal mechanism by which a governmental agency authorizes persons who have met specified minimal standards of competency to engage in a given profession or occupation" (Roemer, 1974, p. 26). Such laws can make licensure either mandatory or voluntary. If they are mandatory, they require all persons who practice the occupation or profession in the state to be licensed. If, on the other hand, they are voluntary, an unlicensed person can practice, but he or she cannot claim to be licensed. Voluntary licensure, therefore, can be viewed as a form of *governmental certification* (Roemer, 1974). Most, if not all, licenses issued for speech-language pathologists and audiologists are of the mandatory type.

The requirements for obtaining an occupational license in a state are specified in a statute enacted by that state's legislature. This statute, among other things, establishes a new licensing board for that occupation or assigns it to an existing board. This board, which functions as (or under the auspices of) an administrative agency, has the responsibility for implementing the licensure program mandated by the statute. Its members are unlikely to all be practitioners of the occupation. Consumers of its services are likely to be included. The board is almost always required by the state to be self-supporting, with expenses met by licensing fees. Such fees for a particular occupation can vary considerably from state to state. Their magnitude, in part, would be a function of the number of persons residing in the state who are likely to seek licensure for that occupation—the larger the number of such persons, the lower the fees are apt to be.

The formulation and passage of a state occupational licensing law (particularly one that is mandatory) is likely to cost the practitioners of the occupation (usually through their state association) a great deal, in terms of both time and money. They are likely to have to retain a lobbyist to guide their bill through the legislative process, and they have no guarantee that the lobbyist's efforts will be successful. If they are successful, practitioners will have to pay a license fee. Considering the financial and time investments involved, why would they seek to have their occupation licensed? Several possible reasons are suggested in the following paragraphs.

> *The primary justification for licensure is the protection of the public. Protection of the public has broader implications than physical damage or loss of life. Unless it can be shown that the public needs protection, attempts to secure licensing regulations are not likely to succeed. . . .*
>
> *In addition to the primary justification mentioned above, there are other important reasons for desiring legislation. For example, licensure of a profession is perhaps the most stringent defense against encroachment on its activities by another profession. . . . Further, licensing legislation tends to force rigorous definition of the activity involved. Finally, the economic advantages of licensure to the licensed group have been clearly recognized.* (Governmental regulation, 1969, p. 41)

The fact that the practitioners of an occupation have succeeded in having a state legislature pass a licensure law does not necessarily mean that their involvement with that legislature has ended. They may have to ask it as some future time to change the requirements for licensure so that these requirements are consistent with how practitioners are being trained. (If the legislation itself is "vague," it may be possible for such changes to be made by the licensing board.) They may also have to convince it to not allow their licensure program to terminate. Some states have *sunset laws* under which entities such as occupational licensing boards are terminated at the end of a specified number of years unless the legislature acts to retain them (Survey of sunset laws, 1991). A legislature is unlikely to act to retain an agency unless it can be convinced that the agency is performing an essential function. Obviously, if an occupational licensing board is scheduled to be terminated and the practitioners of that occupation want it to be retained, they are going to have to convince the members of the legislature that it has been performing such a function.

Most states have passed or are seeking to pass licensing laws for speech-language pathologists and audiologists. The requirements tend to parallel those for the ASHA Certificates of Clinical Competence in Speech-Language Pathology and Audiology.

Institutional Licensure
Institutional licensure has existed for more than forty years. Originally, it was concerned almost exclusively with the quality of facilities (e.g., sanitation and fire safety). Under this form of licensure certain aspects of the functioning of an institution (e.g., a nursing home, hospital, or rehabilitation center) are monitored by a government agency; as long as the institution conforms to certain minimum standards, it remains licensed to perform its function. The agency would tend to more concerned about whether its standards were being met than it would about the means by which they were being met. So long as the institution meets them by lawful means, the agency is unlikely to interfere.

There have been attempts since the early 1970s to extend institutional licensure to include regulating the quality of services provided by an institution (Levine, 1978). Although these attempts for the most part have been unsuccessful, they may foreshadow a movement that at some future time could affect the practice of speech-language pathology and audiology. Such a movement could have considerable impact on practitioners in these professions because the agency monitoring hospitals, rehabilitation centers, nursing homes, and other institutions providing clinical speech, language, and/or hearing services is likely to have its focus on the quality of the services provided—that is, whether they meet *minimum* standards with regard to quality. If the speech, language, and hearing services provided by an institution met the agency's minimum standards, it may not be concerned about whether the persons providing them are licensed in a particular manner by the state or certified by their professional association (particularly the latter). The institution, in a sense, would be responsible for establishing qualifications for persons providing the various services that it offers. Such qualifications may or may not conform to those for individual licensure or certification.

Institutional licensure, *if it were adopted*, could have a significant impact on the practice of speech-language pathology and audiology in medical settings. A hospital, for example, may hire a person who has a bachelor's degree with a major in speech-language pathology or audiology to do basic hearing testing. As long as the hospital could demonstrate that the person was capable of doing such hearing testing with results that possessed at least minimally acceptable levels of validity and reliability and that the person would refer cases requiring more sophisticated testing than he or she could provide, the government agency monitoring the institution would be unlikely to be concerned about the fact that the services were being provided by someone who was neither licensed nor certified in audiology. In fact, it is conceivable that the institution would be commended for not using an expensive, "overqualified" person to provide these services.

Most organizations representing health-related professionals are opposed to that aspect of institutional licensure concerned with establishing qualifications for personnel (Levine, 1978). They fear that with the increasing acceptance of the managed care philosophy (see Chapter 9), some institutions may be tempted to reduce costs by hiring practitioners who do not have the appropriate state license or professional certification. Because of the less than enthusiastic reception that the concept of institutional licensure for personnel has received in many professional circles, it is doubtful that it will replace individual licensure or certification in the near future. It is likely, however, to *coexist* with them in a limited form—for example, by enabling institutions to use unlicensed/uncertified paraprofessional for dispensing some "billable" clinical services (see Chapter 10).

Registration

Registration is a form of certification that is administered by a governmental agency. Persons who have completed the training deemed necessary by the agency to function as a practitioner in a particular field have their names listed in a register (file) that is maintained by that agency. A person may be able to become registered by graduating from a training program that is accredited by the agency.

The certificates that speech-language pathologists obtain from state departments of public instruction that allow them to work in public schools can be viewed as a form of registration. They may be registered almost automatically by completing a training program that is accredited by this state agency.

Registration has also been used in another way for regulating the practice of speech-language pathology and audiology. Some states (e.g., Wisconsin) used it as a first step to licensing them after passing a licensure law.

APPROACHES USED TO REGULATE THE PRACTICE OF SPEECH-LANGUAGE PATHOLOGY AND AUDIOLOGY

Our focus in this chapter thus far has been on the motivation for regulating the practice of an occupation and the approaches that have been used for doing so. We will consider here how these approaches have been used for regulating the practice of speech-language pathology and audiology. The information presented here is rather general because the requirements for credentialing in both fields have been and are likely to continue to be revised frequently.

Certification

The professional association that is most actively involved in the clinical certification of speech-language pathologists and audiologists is the American Speech-Language-Hearing Association (ASHA). ASHA has been certifying the clinical competence of practitioners in communicative disorders since the early 1950s. It currently offers two Certificates of Clinical Competence—one in speech-language pathology and one in audiology. Both require an applicant to have a master's or doctoral degree, to have completed a prescribed program of academic and practicum experience in a graduate program accredited by ASHA, to have completed a clinical fellowship year (i.e., an internship), to have agreed to conform to a code of ethics, and to have passed a national examination. Write to the American Speech-Language-Hearing Association for specific information about the requirements for these certificates.

ASHA did not offer *specialty certification* when this chapter was written. However, it was giving serious consideration to doing so, particularly for the management of fluency disorders.

Accreditation

The American Speech-Language-Hearing Association maintains an accreditation program for master's degree training programs in speech-language pathology and audiology. Both a listing of accredited programs and specific information about requirements for accreditation can be obtained from ASHA. The American Speech-Language-Hearing also maintains an accreditation program for professional services programs.

Licensure

Most states require speech-language pathologists and audiologists to be licensed and have established agencies (boards) for this purpose. The specific requirements for licensure (if a state requires it) can be obtained from the state board responsible for administering the program. The requirements for the credential in most states are those for the Certificate of Clinical Competence in Speech-Language Pathology and the Certificate of Clinical Competence in Audiology.

Registration

The certification that a speech-language pathologist must obtain to be employable in the public schools of a particular state can be viewed as a form of registration. (The rationale for viewing it in this manner is presented elsewhere in this chapter.) The requirements for such certification vary widely from state to state. Those for a particular state can be obtained from its department of public instruction.

As mentioned earlier, several states (e.g., Wisconsin) have used registration to regulate the practice of speech-language pathology and audiology for a few years following the passage of a licensing law while the licensing board is being set up and specific requirements for licensure are being established.

LOSS OF A CREDENTIAL

After the competence of a practitioner or a training program has been recognized by the awarding of a credential, it is tempting for them to assume that their new status is permanent. This is not necessarily true! Certification, licensure, registration, and accreditation can be withdrawn for a variety of reasons. Some of the more frequent ones are considered here.

Reasons for Loss of Certification, Licensure, and Registration

Failure to Abide by the Code of Ethics

A requirement for any form of occupational certification, licensure, or registration is agreeing to be ethical in one's interactions with consumers and follow professionals. Unfortunately, the categorization of behavior as ethical or unethical involves a value judgment—there probably is no behavior that would be categorized as either ethical or unethical by most persons under all circumstances. This being the case, how does a governmental agency or a professional association determine whether particular behavior is unethical? They usually do this by operationally defining (Bridgman, 1961) behaving ethically as adhering to a code of ethics. The code of ethics describes a set of behaviors that can occur in interactions between practitioners and consumers and between practitioners and other professionals, some of which are to be regarded as ethical and others as unethical. If a practitioner does something that is *prohibited* by the code of ethics or fails to do something that the code of ethics *requires*, the practitioner can be classified as behaving in an unethical manner and can lose his or her license, certification, or registration. This appears to be one of the main reasons why persons lose their ASHA certification (see Actions of the ethical practice board, 1986, 1988, 1989a, 1989b, 1991). For further information about codes of professional ethics see Chapter 2.

Failure to Maintain Membership in an Association or to Pay Required Fees

Some associations (including the American Speech-Language-Hearing Association) require persons to whom they award certification to either maintain membership in them or to pay an annual fee, which is regarded as their fair share of the costs to the Association of maintaining the certification program. Failure to do so can result in loss of certification. Similarly, failure to pay licensing and registration fees can result in the loss of these credentials.

Failure to Comply with Changes in Requirements

The requirements for a credential are likely to change from time to time. Must persons who already have the credential meet new requirements? The answer to this question depends on whether there is a *grandfather clause* and, if there is one, what it covers. A grandfather clause excuses a person who is already certified, licensed, or registered from having to meet some new requirements. It is unlikely to excuse him or her from having to meet all of them. Such a clause, for example, would be unlikely to excuse someone who has a credential of one of these types from having to comply with a new continuing education requirement.

The Credential Being Terminated

A person may lose a credential because the program under which it was awarded is terminated. A speech-language pathologist or audiologist could lose his or her license in this manner. The licensure laws for speech-language pathologists and audiologists in a number of states were enacted as sunset laws. When a law is enacted in this way, it is automatically repealed after a certain number of years unless the legislature votes to continue it.

Reasons for Loss of Accreditation

A training program can lose its accreditation for several reasons, singly or in combination. One is that it no longer meets the standards under which it was accredited. This can happen if faculty leave and are not replaced by persons who, in the judgment of the accrediting agency, are competent to teach their courses. Another is that the program cannot meet all of the new standards when it is considered for reaccreditation. The accreditation awarded by most organizations, including the American Speech-Language-Hearing Association, is for a finite number of years. If a training program wishes to remain accredited, it must apply for reaccreditation at the end of this period. Programs that lose their accreditation can make the changes needed to meet current standards and reapply.

PROCEDURES USED FOR TAKING AWAY A CREDENTIAL

The procedures that are used by a professional association or governmental agency for taking away the license, registration, or certification of a practitioner or the accreditation of a training program are supposed to be consistent with the concept of *due process* (specifically, procedural due process), which can be viewed as one of the cornerstones of our legal system (Morris, 1984). If due process is being adhered to by such procedures, the person or training program will be informed of the charges that have been made and will be given an opportunity to answer them. This can involve a hearing during which the agency or association and the individual or training program present evidence to a hearing officer supporting their contentions that the credential should and should not be taken away (see Chapter 7 for information about how hearings are structured). Both parties are likely to be represented by attorneys. Following presentation of the evidence, the hearing officer (who is supposed to be unbiased) decides whether the *preponderance of evidence* supports the charges made by the agency or association. If in his or her judgment the preponderance of evidence supports the charges that were made, the hearing officer can order that the credential be taken away or a lesser penalty if he or she felt that the charges were not serious enough to warrant such action.

A person can appeal the decision of a hearing officer if he or she believes that it was not an appropriate one. At least one level of appeal is usually possible within the agency or association that conducted the hearing. If the person remains dissatisfied after exhausting all internal possibilities for appeal, he or she can initiate a civil suit against the agency or association in an appropriate state or federal court.

It may be possible for charges to be answered without the need for a formal hearing. The association or agency can present the person or program with a written statement of the charges and ask that he, she, or the program *show cause* (in writing) why the credential should not be taken away. If it is obvious from the response that the charges lack merit, the matter can be resolved without a hearing. The American Speech-Language-Hearing Association has used this approach in its clinical certification and accreditation programs.

Write to the American Speech-Language-Hearing Association for information about its appeals procedures. Information about those of state credentialing agencies can be obtained from them.

REFERENCES

Actions of the Ethical Practice Board (1986). *Asha,* 28 (7), 51.
Actions of the Ethical Practice Board (1988). *Asha,* 30 (1), 59.
Actions of the Ethical Practice Board (1989a). *Asha,* 31 (9), 47.
Actions of the Ethical Practice Board (1989b). *Asha,* 31 (11), 59.
Actions of the Ethical Practice Board (1991). *Asha,* 33 (1), 68.
Bridgman, P. W. (1961). *The Logic of Modern Physics.* New York: Macmillan.
Governmental regulation: A statement by the American Speech and Hearing Association. (1969). *Asha,* 11, 39–43.
Levine, L. B. (1978). Institutional licensure versus individual licensure. *Journal of Allied Health,* 7, 109–114.
Lum, J. (1979). Reference groups and professional socialization. In M. Hardy & M. E. Conway (Eds.), *Role Theory: Prospectives for Health Professionals.* Englewood Cliffs, NJ: Prentice Hall.
Morris, W. O. (1984). *Revocation of Professional Licenses by Governmental Agencies.* Charlottesville, VA: The Michie Company.
Roemer, R. (1974). Trends in licensure, certification, and accreditation: Implications for health-manpower education in the future. *Journal of Allied Health,* 3, 26–33.
Rottenberg, S. (1968). Licensing, occupational. In D. L. Sills (Ed.), *International Encyclopedia of the Social Sciences, Volume 9.* New York: Macmillan and Free Press, pp. 283–285.
Silverman, F. H., & Moulton, R. (1997). First class clinical services are possible in a developing country: Speech, language, and hearing in the Gaza Strip. *American Journal of Speech-Language Pathology,* 6 (2), 5–7.
Standards for accreditation of educational programs. (1990). *Asha,* 32 (6), 93–94, 100.
Standards for federal funding. (1972). *Asha,* 14, 546–550.
Survey of sunset laws. (1991). *Governmental Affairs Review,* 12 (3), 15.
White, S. C. (1986). Licensure and third party reimbursement. *Asha,* 28 (6), 36.

▶ 4

Contractual Relationships with Clients and Others

It is almost impossible to be completely self-sufficient in our society. We have to rely on others to provide almost all of the goods and services that we consume. This inescapable reliance on others has several implications. First, it means we must have a way to guarantee that persons who promise to provide us with goods and services do what they promise. And second, it means we must have a way to guarantee that those who keep their promises will receive what they were promised for doing so (which is usually money). The legal instrument that we use in our society for doing both is the *contract*. Without a legal way to enforce promises, a society such as ours in which we must rely on others to satisfy most of our needs would be impossible.

We are continually entering into contracts in both our personal and professional lives. We often are not consciously aware of doing so because we tend to view contracts as written documents that must be signed to be enforceable. A contract does not have to be written to be enforceable. Under certain circumstances oral promises (both direct and implied) and those that are indicated by nonverbal behavior are enforceable as contracts. Also, some written documents that are labeled contracts are not enforceable. Hence, some promises that appear to be enforceable as contracts are not and others that do not appear to be enforceable as contracts are. Since we cannot avoid entering into contracts, we must be able to recognize when we are doing so and be knowledgeable about what the implications are of doing so. My overall objective in this chapter is to increase your level of awareness and understanding of both, particularly as they relate to your functioning as a speech-language pathologist or audiologist.

EVENTS THAT CAN RESULT IN THE CREATION OF A CONTRACT

A contract is an *enforceable promise*. It is described in the authoritative work, *Restatement of the Law: Contracts*, in the following manner: "A contract is a promise for the breach of which the law gives a remedy, or the performance of which the law in some way recognizes as a duty" (1973, p. 5). Thus, a contract is a promise (or a set of promises) that a court is likely to enforce if it is asked to do so. The qualifier "is likely" was used here because the courts do not always do what they would be expected to do. Also, the phrase "if it is asked to do so" was added because a court cannot become involved in the enforcement of a contract unless the person to whom the promise was made that was not kept initiates a civil suit. The threat of such a suit, incidentally, may be enough to motivate a person to do what he or she promised. The reason is that it would be expensive for him or her to be a defendant in a breach-of-contract suit, particularly one that is likely to be successful.

Contracts have also been defined as *enforceable agreements*. When people enter into a contractual relationship, they usually agree to do certain things for each other. For example, an audiologist agrees to test a child's hearing, and the parents or an insurance company agree to pay him or her a certain amount of money for performing this service. The word "agreement" sometimes is substituted for the word "contract" in written contracts.

What role does contract law play in our legal system? The laws that make up our legal system impose restrictions and obligations on our behavior. These restrictions and obligations are of two types: involuntary and voluntary. By residing in the United States, we agree to obey its municipal, state, and federal laws—which are laws of the first type. Our acceptance of the restrictions and obligations they impose on us is not voluntary.

The second type of law that imposes restrictions and obligations on our behavior we voluntarily agree to obey. These laws are created by private individuals rather than legislatures or government agencies. They are private rather than public laws. They can impose restrictions and obligations on the behavior of only a relative small number of persons—often as few as two. They do not duplicate public laws but supplement them. Contract law, which is of this type, provides a mechanism for imposing restrictions and obligations on certain interactions between people that are not regulated by public law—those involving promises.

Contracts are private laws and, like public ones, they are enforced by the courts. The courts have established rules for creating contracts and one that is fabricated in a manner that is consistent with these rules is highly likely to be enforced by them. Consequently, you need to be aware of these rules in order to understand how certain of your actions can intentionally or unintentionally result in the creation of a contract. Some of the more important of these rules will be dealt with in this chapter, particularly those that pertain to *three events* the occurrence of which produce a contract that is likely to be enforced by a court: (1) the making of an *offer*, or promise, (2) the *acceptance* of the offer, and (3) the exchange of *consideration* by the parties—that is, the voluntarily relinquishing of something by each party (e.g., time or money).

The Offer (Promise)

The first event that must occur for a contract to be created is the *making of an offer*. A speech-language pathologist, for example, offers an adult stutterer therapy. The person who makes the offer is referred to as the *offeror* and the person to whom it is made is referred to as the *offeree*. Consequently, the speech-language pathologist in this example would be the offeror and the adult stutterer would be the offeree.

The offer-making process almost always involves the offeror conveying to the offeree (1) what he or she will do for the offeree and (2) what he or she expects in return from the offeree. The word "conveying" was used here rather than "saying" and/or "writing" because an offer can be communicated without the use of spoken or written language. It can be conveyed by implication. Thus, "A promise may be stated in words either oral or written, or may be inferred wholly or partially from conduct" (*Restatement of the Law: Contracts*, 1973, p. 12). The following is an example of a situation in which an offer is conveyed without words:

> *A [letter designates a person], on passing a market, where he has an account, sees a box of apples marked "5 cts. each." A picks up an apple,*

holds it up so that a clerk of the establishment sees the act. The clerk nods, and A passes on. A has promised to pay five cents for the apple. (Restatement of the Law: Contracts, 1973, pp. 12–13)

Similarly, a hard-of-hearing adult who seeks and accepts a hearing aid evaluation from an audiologist conveys to that audiologist by implication a promise to pay him or her (or have a third party do so) a reasonable fee for the evaluation. The presumption in our society is that people are willing to pay a reasonable fee for professional services they ask for and receive.

Theoretically, it should be a relatively easy task to determine whether an offer has been made. All one should have to establish is whether a promise was conveyed from offeror to offeree by words, or by implication, or by some combination of the two. Unfortunately, this may not be an easy task. It depends on what an objective observer (i.e., "reasonable person") would have perceived to be the *intent* of the offeror when he or she said, or wrote, or did what could be construed as an offer. According to Fisher:

Whether an offer has been made depends on intent—the objective intent of a reasonable man observing the actions claimed to constitute the offer. It is not the subjective intent of the offeror that controls the determination of whether an offer has been made (1977, p. 418).

Thus, when attempting to determine whether an offer has been made, a judge would consider if a *reasonable person* hearing or seeing the words or observing the actions that are claimed to have conveyed the offer would conclude that an offer had been made. If the judge feels that a *reasonable person* would have been likely to perceive those words and/or actions as conveying an offer, he or she probably will rule that the intent was to make an offer. On the other hand, if the judge feels that a *reasonable person* would have been unlikely to perceive those words and/or actions as conveying an offer, he or she probably will rule that they do not constitute an offer.

An offer should be as specific and unambiguous as possible. The more specific and unambiguous an offer, the more likely both offeror and offeree will agree on what is being proposed, that is, the obligations they will be expected to assume if the offer is accepted. Also, if an offer is accepted and becomes a contract, a court will have less difficulty determining whether the contract has been breached (violated) if the language meets these criteria.

It is particularly important that when a speech-language pathologist or audiologist offers clinical services to a communicatively handicapped person that the person and/or the family understands that the offer does not promise (guarantee) a cure or a specific level of improvement. All that can be promised (guaranteed) is that the speech-language pathologist or audiologist will attempt to help the person reduce the severity of his or her communicative disorder for as long a period as it is reasonable to expect significant improvement to be possible. A court would be unlikely to view the failure to significantly reduce the severity of a person's communicative disorder as a *breach of contract* if a reasonable attempt was made to reduce its severity. However, a court would be likely to view it as a breach of contract if clinical services were being provided when there was little or no hope for significant improvement. The possible exception would be the person or family, after being informed that the prognosis for further improvement was extremely poor, giving their *informed consent* to therapy services being continued (see the discussion of informed consent in Chapter 12). Furthermore, providing a client with clinical services when there is little or no hope for improvement without his or her or the family's informed consent would be a violation of the American Speech-Language-Hearing Association's Code of Ethics (see Chapter 2).

An offer must be *formally communicated* before it can be accepted and lead to the formation of a contract. What constitutes formal communication is the use of a medium (such as a letter) that is normally used for communicating such offers. If, for example, you heard "through the grapevine" that you had been awarded a grant for which you had applied, you ordinarily could not sue those awarding it for breach of contract if they changed their mind before formally communicating to you (probably in a letter) an offer of the award.

An offeror usually can withdraw, or terminate, an offer during the period between when it is communicated to the offeree and the offeree formally accepts it. There are a variety of reasons an offeror might do this. One that is particularly relevant to clinical practice is referred to as *lapse of a reasonable time*. A person who is offered clinical services by a speech-language pathologist or audiologist should be given a reasonable period of time to decide whether to accept them. When the services are offered, the prospective client should be told how much time he or she has to accept the offer. If the client does not accept it within this time period, the clinician is no longer obliged to either reserve a slot in the schedule for the person or to provide clinical services and products (e.g., hearing aids) for the fee stated in the offer.

Acceptance of the Offer

The second event that must occur for a contract to be formed is the offer being *accepted* by the offeree. An adult stutterer, for example, accepts a speech-language pathologist's offer of therapy.

If an offeree wishes to accept an offer and thereby establish a contract, how must he or she do it? "Acceptance of an offer is a manifestation of assent to the terms thereof made by the offeree in a manner invited or required by the offer" (*Restatement of the Law: Contracts*, 1973, p. 108). Thus, an offeree can accept an offer—that is, the *totality* of what has been offered—by indicating a desire to do so in the manner specified by the offeror (e.g., by signing a contract). If the offeror does not specify how acceptance should be manifested, then any reasonable mode can be used.

There are two basic ways by which acceptance of an offer can be manifested, or indicated. The first of these is acceptance by *performance*. "Acceptance by performance requires that at least part of what the offer requests be performed or tendered" (*Restatement of the Law: Contracts*, 1973, p. 108). Thus, an offeree can indicate acceptance *without words* by beginning to do what acceptance of the offer would require him or her to do, assuming the offer has not been withdrawn or terminated. An adult stutterer could accept a speech-language pathologist's offer of enrollment in a particular ongoing therapy group by attending one or more sessions of that group. Or an audiologist could accept an offer to screen the hearing of the children enrolled in a private school by beginning to screen their hearing.

The second way acceptance can be manifested is by a *promise*. "Acceptance by a promise requires that the offeree complete every act essential to the making of the promise" (*Restatement of the Law: Contracts*, 1973, p. 108). In this case, an offeree would accept an offer by *promising* to do what is required by the offer. He or she may make the promise in words or other symbols (e.g., manual signs) or may imply the promise by conduct. A speech-language pathologist or audiologist in private practice would be accepting an offer by making a promise when he or she signed a *lease* for an office (the lease being a contract). The promise would include the payment of a certain amount of money to the offeror for rent each month for the duration of the lease.

The courts ordinarily do not interpret an offeree's *silence* (i.e., failure to notify the offeror that he or she does not want to accept the offer) as conveying acceptance. Consequently, if a speech-language pathologist told an adult stutterer that she will assume the stutterer wants to be enrolled in the therapy group unless she is informed to the contrary before the end of the month, she would be on shaky ground. The courts usually will rule that an offer has not been accepted unless the offeree conveys acceptance by performance or by making a promise. One of the few exceptions that speech-language pathologists and audiologists are likely to encounter pertains to delivery of the "main selection" in book clubs. Many of these clubs will send you the main selection *offered* each month if you *fail to notify* them within a specified period of time that you don't want it. Here silence after being offered the main selection is interpreted as indicating acceptance of the offer because you agreed to it being interpreted in this manner when you joined.

The offeree must accept the offer in its *entirety* for a contract to be formed. If an offeree is willing to accept parts of it, he or she can convey to the offeror a statement of the parts that he or she is willing to accept. This statement would be regarded as a *counter offer*. The making of a counter offer terminates the offeror's original offer.

The Consideration Exchanged by the Parties

Acceptance of an offer will only result in the formation of a contract if certain conditions are met. One of the most important is that *consideration* be exchanged by the parties. "Consideration embraces the idea that there should be a voluntary relinquishment of a known right by the respective parties to one another for there to be an enforceable agreement by either of them against the other" (Fisher, 1977, p. 449). The courts tend to view it as only fair that *both* offeror and offeree voluntarily agree to give up something (i.e., to assume an obligation that would not have to be assumed if there were no contract). The courts ordinarily will not enforce a contract in which one or both parties failed to voluntarily relinquish a known right.

What constitutes consideration perhaps can be made clearer by describing the two forms it can take. The first is that the offeree agrees to give up something that belongs to the offeree that could *benefit the offeror*.

For example, a hard-or-hearing person (offeror) offers to buy a hearing aid from an audiologist (offeree) for $500. The audiologist accepts the offer and delivers the hearing aid. The transfer and delivery of the hearing aid constitutes consideration because in exchange for a promise to pay $500 the audiologist has voluntarily relinquished something that he owns (a hearing aid) that should benefit the hard-of-hearing person. The hard-of-hearing person, in turn, would be voluntarily relinquishing something that belongs to him—$500.

The second form that consideration can take is that the offeree in accepting an offer agrees to do something that would be recognized by the courts as having a *detrimental* effect on him or her (i.e., cause the offeree to do something he or she wouldn't choose to do) rather than having a beneficial effect on the offeror. The following example illustrates this form of consideration:

> *A promises B, his nephew aged 16, that A will pay B $1000 when B becomes 21 if B does not smoke before then. B's forbearance to smoke is a performance and if bargained for is consideration for A's promise.* (Restatement of the Law: Contracts, 1973, p. 152)

The phrase *bargained for*, as used here, implies that the money offered was not merely a gift. The assumption is being made that B would have smoked if his uncle hadn't made the offer. Thus, in not smoking he would voluntarily be relinquishing a right. It, of course, could be argued that the uncle was receiving a psychological benefit—that is, not having to cope with a nephew who smokes.

For an act to constitute consideration, what is being relinquished by performing the act must be an *actual* (real) known right. Agreeing to do for someone something that one is required to do by law ordinarily would not constitute consideration. Since we are expected to meet our legal obligations, then doing something we are obliged to do anyway would not constitute relinquishing a known right. Consequently, in the following example there is no act that is likely to be construed by a court as constituting consideration since a police officer has a legal duty to produce evidence.

> *A offers a reward to whoever produces evidence leading to the arrest and conviction of the murderer of B. C produces such evidence in the perfor-*

> *mance of his duty as a police officer. C's performance is not consideration for A's promise.* (Restatement of the Law: Contracts, 1973, p. 157)

If a public school speech-language pathologist made an offer to the parents of a language-handicapped child to include their child in her caseload in exchange for an hourly fee and they accepted, she probably would be unsuccessful in suing the parents for breach of contract if they refused to pay her the money after she did so. The clinician was not relinquishing a right by offering to provide clinical services for the child because her contract with the school district required her to do so.

Events That Can Interfere with the Creation of an Enforceable Contract

There are a number of reasons, other than a problem with consideration, that can lead to the acceptance of an offer not resulting in an enforceable contract. Some of the more common ones will be dealt with briefly in this section. For additional information about them see Corbin (1952), Fisher (1977), and *Restatement of the Law: Contracts* (1973).

The events that can interfere with the creation of an enforceable contract that will be dealt with here include the following: (1) incapacity, (2) fraud, (3) mistake, (4) duress, (5) the offer being unconscionable, (6) illegality, and (7) the contract not being in written form when it was required to be. A court may legally excuse a party to a contract from meeting his or her contractual obligations if it can be established that *there is no contract* because of one or more of these reasons. For the acceptance of an offer to result in the creation of a contract *the assumption has to be made* that the parties have the mental and legal capacity to enter into a contract, that one party is not attempting to commit a fraud on the other, that the offer actually was accepted and the contract reflects the agreement (i.e., it contains no *mistakes* that can influence its interpretation), that the offeree did not accept the offer under duress, and so forth. A court is likely to rule that no contract exists and, consequently, neither party can seek damages (money) for it being breached if the *preponderance of evidence* suggests the existence of one or more of these events. They are of more than academic interest. They can provide you with a legal means to escape contractual obligations. And they can provide someone with whom you have a contract a legal means to do so.

Incapacity

The law requires that a person who is accepting an offer have the *mental capacity* to understand the obligations he or she is assuming for the acceptance to result in the formation of a contract. If it can be established that a person lacks such mental capacity, a court is likely to rule that any contracts he or she enters into are unenforceable.

Several categories of persons are almost always assumed by the courts to lack the mental capacity needed to knowledgeably enter into at least some contractual relationships. These include persons who have not yet reached the *age of majority* (children) and persons who are intoxicated. Also included are persons who have been diagnosed as *mentally ill* or *mentally defective*.

A person usually can escape from having to meet at least some contractual obligations by reason of mental incapacity if one or both of the following can be established:

- he is unable to understand in a reasonable manner the nature and consequences of the transaction, or
- he is unable to act in a reasonable manner in relation to the transaction and the other party has reason to know of his condition. (*Restatement of the Law: Contracts*, 1973, p. 33)

One or both probably could be established for persons diagnosed as moderately or severely mentally retarded or for those diagnosed as senile. It may also be possible to establish one or both for persons who have certain communicative disorders resulting from damage to the central nervous system. It could be argued, for example, that a severe receptive aphasic who accepted an offer was "unable to understand in a reasonable manner the nature and consequences of the transaction." A speech-language pathologist, incidentally, might be asked to testify whether in his or her professional opinion it is likely that a particular receptive aphasic who entered into a contract was able to do so (see Chapter 4).

Mental capacity, as defined by these two criteria, is also of concern to audiologists. It could be argued, for example, that a deaf person who does not speechread well and accepted an oral offer was "unable to understand in a reasonable manner the nature and consequences of the transaction." For an in-depth discussion of the implications of the offeree being deaf on the acceptance of an offer (and, hence, on the creation of a contract), see Section 12 in Meyers' (1968) book, *The Law and the Deaf*.

The courts may be unwilling to allow someone to escape from meeting all contractual obligations because of mental incapacity. They may rule that a person is mentally competent to enter into some contractual relationships but not into others. Also, a person may be unable to avoid meeting contractual obligations because the offeror was unaware of his or her mental condition. Some of the issues involved in determining competency are summarized in the following paragraph from the authoritative work, *Restatement of the Law: Contracts*:

The standard of competency. *It is now recognized that there is a wide variety of types and degrees of mental incompetency. Among them are congenital deficiencies in intelligence, the mental deterioration of old age,* the effects of brain damage caused by accident or organic disease *[emphasis mine], and mental illness evidenced by such symptoms as delusions, hallucinations, delirium, confusion, and depression. Where no guardian has been appointed [by a court], there is full contractual capacity in any case unless the mental disease or defect has affected the particular transaction: a person may be able to understand almost nothing, or only simple or routine transactions, or he may be incompetent only with respect to a particular type of transaction. Even though understanding is complete, he may lack capacity to control his acts in the way that the normal individual can and does control them; in such cases the incapacity makes the contract voidable only if the other party has reason to know of his condition. Where a person has some understanding of a particular transaction which is affected by mental illness or defect, the controlling consideration is whether the transaction in its result is one which a reasonably competent person might have made.* (1973, p. 34)

Fraud

Fraud is "an intentional perversion of truth for the purpose of inducing another in reliance upon it to part with some valuable thing belonging to him or to surrender a legal right . . . " (Black, 1968, p. 788). An offeror committing a fraud would *intentionally* provide false information to the offeree to induce acceptance of an offer. The offeror by behaving in this manner is attempting to *defraud* the offeree.

A person who has been defrauded has several options. He or she can ask a court for a release from the contractual obligations—that is, ask the court to rule that no contract exists. Or the person can force the offeror to live up to the contractual obligations if he or she feels that this would be advantageous to him or her (or disadvantageous to the offeror). A contractual relationship that a person was induced to enter because of fraud may become one from which he or she can derive some benefit because of a change in circumstances. Suppose, for example, an audiologist agrees to screen the employees of a factory at some future time for $5000 after the company *intentionally* leads her to believe that the factory employs fewer people than it does. She finds out about this after signing the contract. When the time comes for her to do the screening, she is told that many of the employees have been laid off. Thus, because of a change in circumstances (i.e., fewer employees to screen) the fee she was promised would be more than adequate to compensate her for doing the screening. A court would be unlikely to release the company from its contractual obligation if asked to do so because it originally intended to defraud the audiologist. A judge, in fact, is apt to view enforcement of the contract as yielding poetic justice!

Mistake

A mistake is an *"unintentional* [italics mine] act, omission, or error arising from ignorance, surprise, . . . or misplaced confidence" (Black, 1968, p. 1152). A mistake made by either the offeror or offeree can result in a contract that one or both parties regard as being unfair.

Our concern here pertains to the impact "of action that has been induced by a mistaken thought" (Corbin, 1952, p. 539) on the enforceability of contracts. An offeree may accept an offer ("action") because he or she misunderstood (was mistaken about) what was being offered. Or the offeror may act on the belief that the offeree has accepted the offer when the offeree did not intend to do so. The offeror's action in such an instance would have been "induced by a mistaken thought." (This type of mistake, incidentally, can be prevented by having a written contract: The offeree by signing the contract indicates unequivocally that he or she wants to accept the offer.) Or a person may make an offer *in jest* that is accepted on the mistaken belief that it is a serious offer. Or an offeree may accept an offer (e.g., sign a contract) on the mistaken belief that the information presented in it is accurate, but the offeror unintentionally included inaccurate information in it. In all of these situations there is a possibility a court would rule that no contract exists because acceptance of the offer did not involve a true "meeting of minds." However, there is no guarantee that a court would rule there is no contract. There are circumstances under which a court is likely to rule that a contract is enforceable regardless of the fact that mistakes were made by the offeror, offeree, or both. You should consult an attorney to determine the likelihood that a court will release you from a contractual obligation that you accepted because of a mistake.

While a court may release you from fulfilling a contractual obligation in which there was no true "meeting of minds," it is unlikely to release you from fulfilling one that you accepted but later found to be *disadvantageous*. The courts expect people to study offers carefully before accepting them (e.g., before signing contracts). While you made a mistake not doing so, a court is unlikely to release you from a contractual obligation for this reason.

Duress

The acceptance of an offer is supposed to be a *voluntary* act. A person is supposed to accept an offer because he or she rightly or wrongly views it as advantageous to do so. If a person accepts an offer because he or she actually or figuratively has "a gun held to his or her head," the courts are likely to rule that the offer was accepted under duress and consequently, the contract is void *unless the offeree wishes it to be enforced*. A person who forces someone to accept an offer may end up outsmarted because the contract may unexpectedly prove to be highly advantageous to the offeree. The offeree can insist on enforcement of the contract in such a case and sue the offeror for breach of contract if he or she fails to do what was promised. Such a situation would be one in which poetic justice prevailed.

The Offer Is Unconscionable

Occasionally, a contract contains a clause (or clauses) that is so unreasonably favorable to the interests of one of the parties that a judge is likely to rule that the clause is unenforceable as it stands. A judge would be unlikely to rule part of a contract unconscionable unless it unequivocally violated his or her sense of fairness. Being unconscionable is something beyond one party's bargaining more successfully and as a result getting a better deal. Judges usually are unwilling to rule parts clauses of contracts unconscionable unless the evidence is overwhelming.

Why would a person accept an offer that has aspects that are unconscionable? The only reason probably would be that he or she had no choice. A person who has a desperate need to borrow money but cannot borrow it from a bank because of a poor credit rating may be forced to borrow it from a loan shark at an extremely high interest rate. In the unlikely event that the loan shark sued the person for breach of contract for failure to pay the exorbitant interest rate agreed to, the judge probably would rule that the interest rate was unconscionable and consequently, the contract was unenforceable in its present form. To make it enforceable, the judge probably would order the interest rate to be reduced to one that he or she considered fair.

Illegality

The courts will not enforce a contract that violates either criminal or civil law—that is, one that would result in the commission of a crime or a tort. (See Chapter 5 for a discussion of torts.)

The Contract Is Not in Written Form

While it certainly is desirable for all contracts to be written, for some types it is *essential*. The courts will not enforce them unless they are written. Included here are contracts for the sale of goods over a certain price and those that take longer than a certain period of time to complete. The amounts for both vary from state to state.

Possible Remedies for a Contract Being Breached

You have two options if a person with whom you have a contract refuses to do all or part of what he or she promised to do in it. The first is to seek an *out-of-court settlement* and the second is to sue for *breach of contract*. Most wronged parties initially seek an out-of-court settlement. If this is not attainable, they consider suing for breach of contract. The reason is that the legal fees for an out-of-court settlement are almost always lower than those for a breach-of-contract suit.

Out-of-Court Settlements

The wronged party before initiating a suit will probably attempt to motivate the breaching party to do what was promised, or return whatever was given as payment for doing what was promised, or to pay an amount of money that would compensate for any losses the wronged party sustained. The wronged party may have an attorney draft and send a letter (on the attorney's letterhead) in which there is a direct or implied threat to sue if the matter is not settled out of court. Or he or she may also threaten to file a complaint with an organization such as the Better Business Bureau if the matter is not resolved in a satisfactory manner. Or he or she may contact the consumer advocate at a local television station and ask him or her to intercede. One or more of these actions may be adequate to motivate the breaching party to "do the right thing." If they aren't adequate, an attorney can be retained to initiate a breach-of-contract suit. Most such suits are settled before they come to trial.

Suits for Breach of Contract

A suit for breach of contract is a civil suit and is conducted in the same manner as any other civil suit. The plaintiff (also referred to as the wronged party, the claimant, the grievant, or the petitioner) may seek any of a number of *remedies* from the courts. The one that plaintiff's seek most often in breach-of-contract suits is *compensatory damages*. This consists of an award of money from the defendant (also referred to as the respondent) that is intended to put the plaintiff in the financial position he or she would have been in if the contract had not been breached.

CONTRACTUAL ASPECTS OF THE CLIENT–CLINICIAN RELATIONSHIP

The client-clinician relationship is, among other things, a contractual relationship. The offeror is the clinician and the offeree is the client or his or her family. The consideration offered by the offeror usually is time and expertise. It could also be a device such as a hearing aid. That offered by the offeree is a promise to pay a fee for services rendered. The offeree may or may not be aware of the amount of this fee when treatment is begun. In some cases the fee is paid (partially or fully) by a third party such as a public school system or a medical insurance program (e.g., Medicare). The offeror *offers* a service to the offeree that he or she *accepts*. The offeree is likely to conclude that the offeror has not breached the contract if the offeree receives from the offeror what he or she *thought* the offeror promised.

One frequent problem is that the client (or his or her family) and the clinician have *different interpretations* of the offer. The client when accepting the offer interprets it to be what he or she *wants* it to be rather than what the clinician *intends* it to be. The offeror and offeree do not have a true "meeting of minds." Aside from the legal implications of this situation, it can adversely affect the therapy process.

One way that clients can misconstrue a clinician's offer is to interpret it as guaranteeing significant improvement. They may assume that the clinician by offering his or her services is *implicitly* promising that therapy will be helpful. The clinician, of course, cannot make such a promise for any of several reasons, including the fact that it would violate the ASHA Code of Ethics (see Chapter 2). It is crucial, therefore, that both the client and his or her family understand *before* therapy is initiated that improvement cannot be guaranteed. However, they should be given some estimate of the likelihood that it will be helpful—that is, a statement concerning the prognosis for improvement.

Another way that a client and/or his or her family can misconstrue a clinician's offer is by assuming that the responsibility for the client's improving is completely, or almost completely, the clinician's. They may expect the clinician to do things to the client that will cause the client to change in the manner they desire. Considering the nature of the therapy process, such an assumption is not realistic. Speech-language pathologists and audiologists almost always attempt to help their clients help themselves. The client is expected to assume an active rather than a passive role. It is crucial, therefore, that when therapy is offered, the client and the family be informed as specifically as possible about what the client would be expected to do. Clients should be told that if they are unable or unwilling to do what the clinician expects them to do, they probably will be wasting their time and/or money by accepting the services being offered.

REFERENCES

Black, H. C. (1968). *Black's Law Dictionary* (rev. 4th ed.). St. Paul, MN: West Publishing Company.

Corbin, A. L. (1952). *Corbin on Contracts*. St. Paul, MN: West Publishing Company.

Fisher, B. D. (1977). *Introduction to the Legal System* (2nd ed.). St. Paul, MN: West Publishing Company.

Meyers, L. J. (1968). *The Law and the Deaf*. Washington, DC: Vocational Rehabilitation Administration.

Restatement of the Law: Contracts. St. Paul, MN: American Law Institute. (Copyright 1973 by the American Law Institute. All quotations reprinted with permission of the American Law Institute.)

▶ 5

Malpractice and Other Torts

Persons within our society have an obligation, recognized by the courts, to not act in ways that will harm others physically or mentally nor their reputation or property. They have this obligation regardless of whether there are laws that specifically prohibit actions that would do so. Ignoring this obligation can result in *tort litigation*. If a speech-language pathologist, for example, were to contribute to a delay is a diagnosis of laryngeal cancer by not insisting that a patient be examined by indirect laryngoscopy before beginning voice therapy, he or she could sue the clinician for the tort of *malpractice*. Or if a clinician were to use corporal punishment to discipline a child, the child's parents could sue the clinician for the tort of *battery*. Or if the use of response-contingent "time out" caused a child a great deal of mental distress, the child's parents could sue the clinician for the tort of *infliction of mental distress*. Or if a clinician told a potential patient of a practitioner that he or she was incompetent or unethical, the practitioner could sue the clinician for the tort of *slander*. Of course, a person who initiates such tort litigation may lose. Some factors that can influence the likelihood that he or she will win are discussed elsewhere in this chapter.

My objective in this chapter is to acquaint you with the law of torts as it relates to clinical practice in speech-language pathology and audiology. I will begin by describing some of the basic characteristics of torts. Next, I'll describe some of the types of torts against which clinicians should be proactive in protecting themselves, including the negligence tort of *mal-*

practice. We will then consider how a clinician would function who wanted to minimize the likelihood of becoming involved in tort-related litigation. Finally, several types of liability insurance will be described that offer a clinician some protection if sued.

WHAT IS A TORT?

There appears to be almost universal agreement among writers of books on torts that the term "tort" is a difficult one to define (Prosser, 1971). One reason is that some of the acts that the courts have classified as torts seem to have little in common with others. Another reason is that the courts through their decisions have classified acts as torts that they previously refused to classify as torts. Some of these reversals could not have been predicted from definitions of the term "tort" that existed at the time (Prosser, 1971).

Courts create torts—acts become torts when they are classified as such by the courts. This is one reason why it has been difficult to arrive at a satisfactory definition of the term "tort." Existing definitions appear to have been based, at least in part, on explanations that judges gave in their decisions for why they classified something as a tort. However, the reasons that the judges gave may not have been their real reasons for doing so. They may merely have been ones that the judges regarded as being "politically correct."

While existing definitions of the term "tort" are not completely satisfactory, they do shed some light on the characteristics of acts that the courts have classified as torts. The following are a sampling of such definitions:

- A private or civil wrong or injury. A wrong independent of contract. (Black, 1968, p. 1660)
- A legal wrong committed upon the person or property independent of contract. It may be either (1) a direct invasion of some legal right of the individual; (2) the infraction of some public duty by which special damage accrues to the individual; (3) the violation of some private obligation by which like damage accrues to the individual. In the former case, no special damage is necessary to entitle the party to recover. In the two latter cases, such damage is necessary (Black, 1968, pp. 1660–1661)

- A tort is a breach of a duty (other than a contractual or quasi-contractual duty) which gives rise to an action for damages. (Prosser, 1971, p. 1)
- A tort is an act or omission which unlawfully violates a person's right created by the law, and for which the appropriate remedy is a common law action for damages by the injured person. (Prosser, 1971, p. 2)
- Broadly speaking, a tort is a civil wrong, other than breach of contract, for which the court will provide a remedy in the form of an action for damages. (Prosser, 1971, p. 2)
- It might be possible to define a tort by enumerating the things it is not. It is not a crime, it is not breach of contract, it is not necessarily concerned with property rights or problems of government, but it is the occupant of a large residuary field remaining if these are taken out of the law. (Prosser, 1971, p. 2)
- Included under the head of torts are a miscellaneous group of civil wrongs, ranging from simple, direct interference with person, such as assault, battery and false imprisonment, or with property, as in the case of trespass or conversion, up through various forms of negligence, to disturbances of intangible interests, such as those in good reputation, or commercial or social advantage. These wrongs have little in common and appear at first glance to be entirely unrelated to one another . . . and it is not easy to discover any general principle upon which they may all be based, unless it is the obvious one that *injuries are to be compensated and anti-social behavior is to be discouraged* [italics mine]. (Prosser, 1971, p. 3)
- . . . the function and purpose of the law of torts. Contract liability is imposed by the law for the protection of a single, limited interest, that of having the promises of others performed. Quasi-contractual liability is created for the prevention of unjust enrichment of one man at the expense of another, and the restitution of benefits which in good conscience belong to the plaintiff. The criminal law is concerned with the protection of interests common to the public at large, as they are represented by the entity which we call the state; and it accomplishes its ends by exacting a penalty from the wrongdoer. *There remains a body of law which is directed toward the compensation of individuals, rather than the public, for losses which they have suffered in respect of all their legally recognized interests, rather than one interest only, where the law considers that compensation is required* [italics mine]. This is the law of torts. (Prosser, 1971, pp. 5–6)

- The entire history of the development of tort law shows a continuous tendency to recognize as worthy of legal protection interests which previously were not protected at all. . . . It is altogether unlikely that this tendency to give protection to hitherto unprotected interests and to extend a greater protection to those now frequently protected has ceased. (*Restatement of the Law: Torts*, 1965–1979, Section 1)

Several general characteristics of torts are indicated in these definitions. First, torts are *civil wrongs* rather than criminal wrongs. They are not crimes. They are wrongs against individuals rather than against society. Consequently, in a lawsuit involving a tort the plaintiff (claimant, grievant, petitioner) is a person, or group of persons, rather than a governmental unit (e.g., the state).

A second characteristic of a tort is that it is a civil wrong for which a court is willing to provide a *remedy*. The remedy is likely to be an award of money (i.e., *damages*) to compensate the injured party for the harm done to him or her or an order to the defendant (respondent) to cease doing whatever he or she is doing that is causing the plaintiff harm (i.e., an *injunction*).

The willingness of the courts to provide a remedy for some civil wrongs (such as libel and negligence) is well established. For others, it may be necessary to initiate a lawsuit to determine whether a court is willing to provide a remedy—that is, to establish whether the court is willing to classify a particular type of wrong as a tort.

A third characteristic of a tort is that it is a civil wrong that is not the breach of a contract. The breach of a contract is a civil wrong resulting from the failure of a person to do what he or she voluntarily promised to do. (See Chapter 4 for further information about contracts.) The same act performed by a person who had not voluntarily agreed to refrain from doing it (by entering into a contract) probably would not be regarded by a court as a civil wrong (assuming that a judge would not regard it as a tort). On the other hand, one is expected by society to refrain from engaging in acts that can harm others. Consequently, the breach of a contract differs from a tort in that the former involves the breaking of a promise that one has made voluntarily to a specific person (or a relatively small group of people) and the latter involves the breaking of a promise that one was required by "law" to make to all persons with whom one interacts.

A fourth characteristic of a tort is that it results from interference with the realization of a legally protected desire. The realization of certain desires is considered by the courts to be of such social importance that they are obliged to discourage persons from thwarting them. They do this by imposing *liability* (e.g., damages) on those who interfere with the realization of these desires either *intentionally* or through *negligence*.

What types of desires have the courts been willing to protect from being thwarted? There are many (see the multivolume work, *Restatement of the Law: Torts*, 1965–1979), including the following:

- The desire for *bodily security*—the desire not to be physically harmed or even being touched by another without your permission, either intentionally or through negligence (e.g., malpractice).
- The desire for a *reputation* that is commensurate with your behavior—the desire not to have your reputation damaged by someone's saying or writing something about you that is untrue.
- The desire for your *property* to be secure—the desire for your property not to be damaged, used, or even touched by another without your permission, either intentionally or through negligence.
- The desire for your *mental state* to be secure—the desire not to have your intellectual or emotional status harmed by another, either intentionally or through negligence.

Some of the torts that can result from these types of desires being thwarted are described in the next section.

TYPES OF TORTS

Most actions that are classifiable as torts can be assigned to one of three categories: negligence torts, intentional torts, or strict liability. This section describes some professionally relevant torts that are representative of those in each category.

Negligence Torts

Negligence torts involve accidental harm to others. However, not all actions that accidentally harm others are classified by the courts as negligence torts. A court will only classify an action in this way if following four conditions are met:

1. The interest invaded is protected against unintentional invasion.
2. The conduct of the actor is negligent with respect to the other, or to a class of persons within which he is included.

3. The actor's conduct is a legal cause of the invasion.

4. The other has not conducted himself as to disable himself from bringing an action for an invasion. (*Restatement of the Law: Torts, 1965–1979,*
Section 281)

The first and second conditions must be met for the conduct of a person
who is responsible for an accident to be regarded as negligent by the
courts. The third and fourth conditions must be met before a court probably would be willing to award damages for negligent conduct, once it
had been established that it had occurred. If the first two conditions were
met but not the third and fourth, the court might agree that the actor's
conduct was negligent but would not award damages. Consequently, the
attorney for a defendant in a malpractice suit may attempt to prove that
the third and/or fourth condition was not met and, for this reason, damages should not be awarded to the plaintiff.

The courts have been willing to protect a number of interests against
unintentional invasion by reason of carelessness. The following excerpts
from the authoritative *Restatement of the Law: Torts, 1965–1979* indicate
some of the types of negligent acts against which the courts have been
willing to offer protection:

1. . . . acts which are generally regarded as reasonably safe if properly
done, the only danger involved in them lying in the chance that the
actor may be inattentive, incompetent, or unskillful or that he may fail
to make adequate preparation or give adequate warning [Section
297]. When an act is negligent only if done without reasonable care,
the care which the actor is required to exercise to avoid being negligent in the doing of the act is that which a *reasonable man* [italics mine]
in his position, with his information and competence, would recognize as necessary to prevent the act from creating an unreasonable
risk of harm to another [Section 298].

(a) An act may be negligent if it is done without the competence
which a *reasonable man* [italics mine] in the position of the actor
would recognize as necessary to prevent it creating an unreasonable risk of harm to another [Section 299]. Unless he represents
that he has greater or less skill or knowledge, one who undertakes
to render services in the practice of a profession or trade is required to exercise the skill and knowledge normally possessed by

members of that profession or trade in good standing in similar communities [Section 299A].

(b) When an act is negligent when done without reasonable preparation, the actor, to avoid being negligent, is required to make the preparation which a *reasonable man* [italics mine] in his position would recognize as necessary to prevent the act from creating an unreasonable risk of harm to another [Section 300].

2. An act may be negligent if the actor attempts to prevent, or realizes or should realize that it is likely to prevent, another or a third person from taking action which the actor realizes or should realize is necessary for the aid or protection of the other [Section 305]. [Beginning voice therapy before having a client's vocal folds checked for pathology by an otolaryngologist may be viewed by a court as such an act.]

3. An act may be negligent, as creating an unreasonable risk of bodily harm to another, if the actor intends to subject, or realizes or should realize that his act involves an unreasonable risk of subjecting, the other to an emotional disturbance of such a character as to be likely to result in illness or other bodily harm [Section 306].

4. It is negligence to use an instrumentality, whether a human being or a thing, which the actor knows or should know to be so incompetent, inappropriate, or defective, that its use involves an unreasonable risk of harm to others [Section 307]. [The use of students in training or paraprofessionals to provide clinical services without adequate supervision may be viewed by the courts as this type of negligent act.]

For further information about the types of negligent acts referred to in these excerpts as well as other types of negligent acts for which courts have been willing to provide a remedy, see Chapters 12 through 19 in *Restatement of the Law: Torts, 1965–1979*; Bebout's (1986) paper, "The malpractice storm"; Feuer's (1990) book, *Medical Malpractice Law*; Kooper and Sullivan's chapter, "Professional liability: Management and prevention (1986); and Rowland's (1988) paper, "Malpractice in audiology and speech-language pathology."

What standard do the courts use to judge whether the conduct of an actor was negligent? The standard, which is referred to in several of these excerpts, is that of the hypothetical *reasonable man*. A person who does not take the precautions that *a reasonable man in the same position* would be expected to take in order to avoid harming others is likely to be regarded as negligent by a court if someone is harmed by the act: "Unless the actor is a child, the standard to which he must conform to avoid being negligent is that of a reasonable man under like circumstances" (*Restatement of the Law: Torts, 1965–1979*, Section 283).

If the standard of conduct to which you must conform to avoid being negligent is that of a reasonable man under like circumstances, you should be aware of the *qualities* that the courts ascribe to their hypothetical reasonable man. These are summarized as follows in Section 283 of the *Restatement of the Law: Torts*:

> *The words "reasonable man" denote a person exercising those qualities of attention, knowledge, intelligence, and judgment which society requires of its members for the protection of their own interests and the interests of others. It enables those who are to determine whether the actor's conduct is such as to subject him to liability for harm caused thereby, to express their judgment in terms of the conduct of a human being. The fact that this judgment is personified in a "man" calls attention to the necessity of taking into account the fallibility of human beings.*

Deciding whether a person's conduct in a particular situation conforms to what would be expected from a reasonable man in like circumstances may not be easy because it may be unclear how a reasonable man would conduct himself. The attorney for the defendant in a negligence suit is likely to attempt to convince the judge and jury that his or her client's conduct conformed to that of the hypothetical reasonable man and consequently, the second of the four conditions that must be met before a court is supposed to award damages for negligence has not been met.

The third condition is that the actor's (defendant's) conduct be the *legal cause* of the harm to the plaintiff. Being able to demonstrate that you were harmed because of someone's negligence is not sufficient to be awarded damages. You also have to be able to demonstrate that the negligent act that caused you to be harmed is one for which the courts have been willing to award damages—that is, the act has been recognized as a legal cause.

What causes have the courts recognized as legal causes? According to Section 431 of the *Restatement of the Law: Torts*:

The actor's negligent conduct is a legal cause of harm to another if

(a) his conduct is a *substantial factor* [italics mine] in bringing about the harm, and

(b) there is no rule of law relieving the actor from liability because of the manner in which his negligence has resulted in harm.

A defendant's conduct is likely to be considered a substantial factor in bringing about the harm that was done to a plaintiff if a *reasonable man* would be likely to regard it as such. Consequently, a defendant's attorney may argue that while his or her conduct was negligent, it is not reasonable to regard it as being a substantial factor is bringing about the harm that was done to the plaintiff. If the attorney is successful, the plaintiff is unlikely to be awarded damages.

A defendant can be relieved of liability for a particular negligent act if there is a *rule of law* that relieves persons from negligence liability for that act. A physician, for example, may be relieved from negligence liability for complications arising from an emergency tracheotomy performed on a person who probably would have died otherwise if there is a law that prevents physicians from being sued for harm resulting from such emergency procedures.

The fourth and final condition that has to be met before a court is likely to award damages for negligence is that the plaintiff must have conducted himself or herself in a manner that would not disqualify him or her from being awarded them. A plaintiff can be disqualified by acting in a manner that is *below the standard of conduct* that would be reasonable to expect of someone for their own protection. Plaintiffs who do not adequately protect themselves are contributing to the negligence that causes them to be harmed. In some states, if a defendant can prove *contributory negligence* on the part of the plaintiff, this will bar the plaintiff from receiving damages; in other states, contributory negligence does not disqualify the plaintiff from being awarded damages but is considered by the court when deciding the amount of damages to award (*Restatement of the Law: Torts, 1965–1979,* Chapter 17).

What constitutes contributory negligence on the part of a plaintiff? According to the *Restatement of the Law: Torts* (Sections 463 & 464), contributory negligence can be defined as follows:

Contributory negligence is conduct on the part of the plaintiff which falls below the standard to which he should conform for his own protection, and which is a legally contributing cause co-operating with the negligence of the defendant in bringing about the plaintiff's harm. . . . Unless the actor is a child or an insane person, the standard of conduct to which he must conform for his own protection is that of the reasonable man under like circumstances.

The attorney for the defendant in a negligence suit may attempt to prove that the plaintiff did not protect himself or herself as well as a reasonable person should have under the circumstances and consequently, the plaintiff was negligent also.

We have dealt thus far with the general conditions that have be met before an act causing harm to another is likely to be regarded by the courts as a negligence tort. We will now shift our focus to the type of negligence tort about which speech-language pathologists and audiologists are likely to be most concerned—*malpractice.*

Any type of negligent conduct by a professional that causes his or her patient (client) to be harmed either physically or mentally may be regarded by a court as constituting malpractice. As applied to health-care professionals,

the term means, generally, professional misconduct toward a patient which is considered reprehensible either because being immoral in itself or because being contrary to law or expressly forbidden by law.

In a more specific sense it means bad, wrong, or injudicious treatment of a patient, professionally and in respect to the particular disease or injury, resulting in injury, unnecessary suffering, or death of the patient, and proceeding from ignorance, carelessness, want of proper professional skills, disregard of established rules or principles, neglect, or a malicious or criminal intent. (Black, 1968, p. 1111)

Society expects professionals to exercise reasonable care and to possess a standard minimum of special knowledge and ability (Prosser, 1971). The standard minimum ordinarily is that specified in the requirements for the license or certification required for practicing the profession.

While the defendants in the majority of malpractice lawsuits involving health-care practitioners have been physicians, practitioners in almost every health-care field, including speech-language pathology and audiology, have been defendants in such suits (Miller, 1983; Miller & Lubinski, 1986). Almost all health-care practitioners have malpractice insurance because the cost of defending yourself in a malpractice lawsuit can be quite high even if you win (see Liability lawsuits present danger to qualified professionals, says official, 1985). Speech-language pathologists and audiologists who are employed by school systems, hospitals, or other institutions usually get malpractice insurance coverage from their employer. Those who do private practice (full- or part-time) obviously have to purchase their own malpractice insurance. Contact the American Speech-Language-Hearing Association for the names of companies that offer it.

What sort of conduct by a speech-language pathologist or audiologist could result in a malpractice suit? There are a number of scenarios that could result in such a suit, including the following:

- A speech-language pathologist accepts for voice therapy a person who has a hoarse voice and does not insist that he be seen by an otolaryngologist for a laryngeal examination. The person discovers six months later that his hoarseness resulted from laryngeal cancer. He claims that he was harmed because the condition was not diagnosed earlier and that this was due to the speech-language pathologist's negligence in not insisting on his having a laryngeal examination before therapy was begun.
- A speech-language pathologist administers swallowing therapy to an adult who has been diagnosed as having dysphagia. The clinician does not have suctioning equipment in the room that she (or someone else such as a nurse) can use if the person begins to choke. The client chokes on some food during a therapy session and dies. The family sues the speech-language pathologist claiming that she had been negligent by not having suctioning equipment available in the room while doing the swallowing therapy.
- An audiologist inserts an impedance probe into a child's ear without first examining the external canal with an otoscope to make certain that there is no object in the canal that could damage the tympanic membrane if pushed against it. The insertion of the probe results in an object being pushed against the membrane and damaging it. The family sues the audiologist claiming that he or she had been negligent by not examining the canal before inserting the probe.
- A two-year-old child swallowed the battery of a hearing aid that had been prescribed by an audiologist. Surgery was necessary to remove the battery. The parents sue the audiologist claiming that he was negligent by not warning them about the possibility of this occurring.

For other malpractice scenarios that are relevant to our profession, see Kramer and Armbruster (1982) Lowe (1988), and Rowland (1988).

Intentional Torts

Intentional torts result from acts that are *intended* to injure or harm others and/or are morally wrong. They differ from negligence torts in that the harm done to a person is not due to carelessness. If, for example, I tell someone that a particular practitioner is a quack, my intent probably is to damage his or her reputation and, thereby, discourage people from using his or her services. If the person sues me and I am unable to prove—that is, establish by the "preponderance of evidence"—that he or she is incompetent, the court is likely to award the person damages for being *slandered*.

The word *intent*, as used in this context, denotes the actor's awareness that his or her act is likely to have certain consequences. According to Section 8A of the *Restatement of the Law: Torts,*

> *All consequences which the actor desires to bring about are intended.* . . . *Intent is not, however, limited to consequences which are desired. If the actor knows that the consequences are certain, or substantially certain, to result from his act, and still goes ahead, he is treated by the law as if he had in fact desired to produce the result. As the probability that the consequences will follow decreases, and becomes less than substantial certainty, the actor's conduct loses the character of intent, and becomes mere recklessness.* . . . *As the probability decreases further, and amounts only to a risk that the result will follow, it becomes ordinary negligence.*

Consequently, people can be held accountable not only for desired consequences of their acts, but also for others that they know are likely to occur.

What *types of acts* are the courts likely to classify as intentional torts? Some that can occur while you are interacting with clients and their families are described briefly here. For further information about these and others, see Prosser (1971) and *Restatement of the Law: Torts, 1965–1979.*

Invasion of Privacy

A right to privacy—to be let alone—has been recognized by the courts. Interference with this right can result in litigation for the tort known as *in-*

vasion of privacy. In a clinical context, such litigation can result from releasing reports or other information about a client without his or her written consent, using photographs of a client in clinic promotional material without written consent, writing about the client in published case studies in a way that he or she is recognizable without such consent, or allowing someone to view a client's clinic sessions through a one-way mirror without consent.

Defamation

If someone says or writes something false and malicious about you that injures your reputation, you may be successful if you sue that person for either the tort of libel or of slander. If the false and malicious statements were communicated in *written or printed* form, you ordinarily would sue for *libel*; if they were communicated in *oral* form, you ordinarily would sue for *slander*. The law in this area is quite complex, and you would have to consult an attorney to determine whether the courts would be likely to award you sufficient damages (money) to make a suit for defamation (i.e., slander or libel) worthwhile. You could conceivably win a defamation suit and be awarded only *nominal damages*—for example, one dollar.

Unfortunately, not every statement that someone makes about you that you regard as being false and malicious is likely to be viewed by the courts as being libelous or slanderous. Under what circumstances would a court be likely to view such a statement in this way? According to Prosser,

> defamation is—that which tends to injure "reputation" in the popular sense; to diminish the esteem, respect, goodwill or confidence in which the plaintiff is held, or to excite adverse, derogatory or unpleasant feelings or opinions against him. It necessarily, however, involves the idea of disgrace [emphasis mine]. (1971, p. 729)

While the statement that an audiologist is sympathetic to the use of sign rather than speech by deaf persons is likely to elicit negative feelings against him or her in the minds of those who are against their use of sign and may even diminish the audiologist in their esteem, a court would be unlikely to consider it defamatory. A *reasonable person* would be unlikely to consider that it reflects upon the audiologist's character and consequently, would cause him or her to be disgraced. On the other hand, a statement that an audiologist is unethical would be likely to be viewed by a court as defamatory since a reasonable man would be likely to conclude that it does reflect on the audiologist's character and consequently, could cause him or her to be disgraced.

A professional's reputation determines to a considerable extent how successfully he or she is likely to be financially and otherwise. Therefore, the courts have recognized that they have a special responsibility to protect professionals against false and malicious statements about their capacity and professional conduct. Speech-language pathologists and audiologists not only risk lawsuits by making false and malicious statements about other professionals, but they also violate the Code of Ethics of the American Speech-Language-Hearing Association by doing so (see Chapter 2).

Infliction of Mental Distress

If someone says or does something that causes you *severe* mental (emotional) distress, you can seek relief from a court. The relief you would seek might be an *injunction* that would order the person to stop saying or doing what is causing you distress or it might be *damages* to compensate you for the harm that the distress has done.

The word "severe" was italicized in the preceding paragraph because the courts are unlikely to compensate you for most things that people say or do that make you upset. The courts assume that a *reasonable person* should be able to keep from becoming overly upset by most things that people say or do. Furthermore, if the courts were willing to award damages for insults and most other things that people regard as irritating, there probably would be so many lawsuits that the civil courts would become hopelessly bogged down.

For what types of stress-inducing conduct are the courts likely to offer relief? According to Section 46 of the *Restatement of the Law: Torts*:

> one who by extreme and outrageous conduct intentionally or recklessly causes severe emotional distress to another is subject to liability for such emotional distress, and if bodily harm to the other results from it, for such bodily harm.

Consequently, for conduct that causes emotional distress to be compensable, it would have to be such that the hypothetical reasonable person would view it a *extreme and outrageous*. The courts are likely to consider the following comment from Section 46 of the *Restatement of the Law: Torts* as a guideline when deciding whether conduct has been extreme and outrageous:

> Extreme and outrageous conduct. *The cases thus far decided have found liability only where the defendant's conduct has been extreme and outrageous. It has not been enough that the defendant has acted with an intent which is tortuous or even criminal, or that he has intended to inflict emotional distress, or even that his conduct has been characterized by "malice," or a degree of aggravation which would entitle the plaintiff to punitive damages for another tort. Liability has been found only where the conduct has been so outrageous in character, and so extreme in degree, as to go beyond all possible bounds of decency, and to be regarded as atrocious, and utterly intolerable in a civilized community. Generally, the case is one in which the recitation of the facts to an* average member of the community *[emphasis mine] would arouse his resentment against the actor, and lead him to exclaim, "Outrageous!"*

One technique that speech-language pathologists and audiologists have used with communicatively handicapped children and adults that could be viewed by the average member of the community as extreme and outrageous is response-contingent punishment, such as administration of electric shocks. The average member of your community (whose views would reflect the attitudes of most juries) is likely to consider giving electric shocks to handicapped children to be outrageous. It is essential, therefore, that written consent be obtained from clients or their families before using any technique that could be viewed by "the average member of your community" in this way. The rationale for using the technique and the risks involved should be explained to the client's family and possibly to the client so that the written consent procured is likely to be viewed by a court as having been *informed consent*.

Assault

If others by their actions and/or words caused you to become apprehensive about being harmed by them (that is, if they threaten to harm you), you can sue them for the tort of assault. Assault does not involve actual undesired physical contact, only the *threat* of such contact. This tort is actually a special case of *infliction of mental distress*, the mental distress being caused by a threat of physical harm.

Battery

If someone intentionally touched you without your permission (even if the contact resulted in no physical injury such as would ordinarily be the case for a kiss), you could sue them for the tort of battery. The courts will protect your right to freedom from intentional and unpermitted physical contacts (Prosser, 1971).

This tort differs from assault in that there is actual physical contact. If someone both made you apprehensive about being physically harmed and intentionally physically touched you, you could sue them for both *assault and battery*.

Since plaintiffs in a suit for battery do not have to prove that they were physically harmed, only that they were touched without permission, this tort could have implications for clinicians. Touching a client lightly on the arm without permission could lead to being sued for battery as could removal of his or her hearing aid without permission (Rowland, 1988). While few clients are likely to even consider initiating such a suit, a clinician should be aware of the possibility and refrain from touching a client who seems like the "suing kind." Obviously such a suit (whether it had any merit) could seriously damage a clinician's reputation.

Strict Liability

In both negligence torts and intentional torts, a plaintiff is awarded damages because the conduct of the defendant was in some way *faulty*. When suing for these types of torts, the plaintiff must establish that the negligence or purposeful conduct of the defendant was responsible for the harm done to him or her before a court will award damages.

The fact that the plaintiff was harmed by the defendant is sufficient in some circumstances to cause the court to award the plaintiff damages. This is referred to as *strict liability*. According to Prosser,

> . . . the last hundred years have witnessed the overthrow of the doctrine of "never any liability without fault," even in the legal sense of departure from reasonable standards of conduct. It has seen a general acceptance of the principle that in some cases the defendant may be held liable, although he is not only charged with no moral wrongdoing, but has not even departed in any way from a reasonable standard of intent or care. . . . This new policy frequently has found expression when the defendant's activity is unusual and abnormal in the community, and the danger

which it threatens to others is unduly great—and particularly where the danger will be great even though the enterprise is conducted with every possible precaution (1971, p. 494)

Consequently, an industrial firm could be held responsible for hearing losses of its employees that resulted from being exposed to high levels of noise on the job even though the firm took "every possible precaution."

TORT LITIGATION AND THE CLINICIAN

Speech-language pathologists and audiologists, like practitioners in other health-related professions, are at risk for tort-related litigation. Since such litigation can have a detrimental impact on both your finances and reputation, everything possible should be done to minimize this risk. You can do this by heightening your awareness of events that can occur in your interactions with clients and their families that could lead to such litigation and then taking appropriate precautions. If you are uncertain about the adequacy of any of the precautions you are taking, you would be wise to consult with an attorney.

The risk of becoming a defendant in tort litigation can be minimized, but it cannot be entirely eliminated. It is important, therefore, to carry adequate *professional liability insurance* (see Miller, 1983; Miller & Lubinski, 1986). It usually will be provided by your employer unless your relationship to him or her is one of *independent contractor* (see Chapter 16 for a discussion of this relationship). If it is not provided by your employer or you are in private practice, contact the American Speech-Language-Association for information about vendors.

REFERENCES

Bebout, M. (1986). The malpractice storm. *Hearing Journal*, 39 (2), 7–12.

Black, H. C. (1968). *Black's Law Dictionary* (Rev. 4th ed.). St. Paul, MN: West Publishing Company.

Feuer, W. W. (1990). *Medical Malpractice Law*. Irvine, CA: LawPrep Press.

Kooper, R., & Sullivan, C. A. (1986). Professional liability: Management and prevention. In K. G. Butler (Ed.), *Prospering in Private Practice*. Rockville, MD: Aspen.

Kramer, M. B., & Armbruster, J. M. (Eds.) (1982). *Forensic Audiology*. Baltimore, MD: University Park Press.

Liability lawsuits present danger to qualified professionals, says official (1985). *Asha*, 27 (6), 9–10.

Lowe, R. G. (1988). Are audiologists guilty of malpractice if they do not recommend binaural amplification? *Asha*, 30 (11), 39–40.

Miller, T. D. (1983). *Professional Liability in Speech-Language Pathology and Audiology: Unprofessional Conduct and Unethical Practice*. Unpublished doctoral dissertation, State University of New York at Buffalo.

Miller, T. D., & Lubinski, R. (1986). Professional liability in speech-language pathology and audiology. *Asha*, 28 (6), 45–47.

Prosser, W. L. (1971). *Law of Torts* (4th ed.). St. Paul, MN: West Publishing Company.

Restatement of the Law: Torts (2nd ed.). St. Paul, MN: American Law Institute. (Copyright 1979 by the American Law Institute. All quotations reprinted with permission of the American Law Institute.)

Rowland, R. C. (1988). Malpractice in audiology and speech-language pathology. *Asha*, 30 (1), 45–48.

▶ 6

Influencing Legislation

The Code of Ethics of the American Speech-Language-Hearing Association requires speech-language pathologists and audiologists to "hold paramount the welfare of persons served professionally." Furthermore, it requires them to "expand services to persons with speech, language, and hearing problems." These injunctions imply that speech-language pathologists and audiologists have a responsibility to persons who are communicatively impaired that extends beyond their own caseloads. This responsibility includes doing everything possible to insure that persons requiring speech, language, or hearing services are able to receive them.

One of the main reasons why persons who are communicatively impaired may not receive needed services is *lack of funding*. The clinical services received by the majority of such persons are not paid for directly by them or their families. They are paid for by a *third party*, most often a governmental administrative agency. These agencies (including local school boards, state departments of public instruction, and the federal Social Security Administration) are able to provide the funding because they have been allocated funds for the purpose by municipal, state, or federal legislatures. Such legislatures have the ability to maintain a given level of funding for speech, language, and hearing services, to increase this level of funding, or to reduce it. The level of funding they allocate for such services is partially determined by the arguments that are presented to them for increasing, reducing, or maintaining the existing level. These arguments are presented to them to persons functioning as *lobbyists*.

After 1972, the frequency with which speech-language pathologists and audiologists functioned as lobbyists at the federal level for persons who are communicatively impaired increased dramatically. This increase in activity at the federal level was due mainly to the creation in that year of the American Speech-Language-Hearing Association's *Congressional Action Contact (CAC) Network* (Congressional Action Contact Network Handbook, 1991). A member of the Association is assigned to each member of Congress (each senator and each representative) to lobby the legislator on bills that are or will be under consideration. The member assigned is a constituent of the legislator. Some state associations now maintain similar networks for lobbying members of their legislature. "All state associations need member support to assist in [legislative and regulatory] grass-roots activities" (Browne, 1991, p. 40).

I have two objectives in this chapter. The first is to increase your awareness of the need for lobbying "to promote the welfare of the persons whom we serve professionally" and the second is to provide you with some practical information on how to promote their welfare by lobbying. Hopefully, the information presented will cause you to give serious consideration some time in the future to the possibility of participating in ASHA's Congressional Action Contact (CAC) Network or a comparable network maintained by your state association. I've been involved with ASHA's CAC Network since its inception and believe wholeheartedly that the time I've invested has been well spent.

WHAT IS A LOBBYIST?

Anyone who *consciously* attempts to influence the activities (particularly the votes) of a legislator can be regarded as being a lobbyist. The legislator being lobbied may be a member of the United States Congress or of a state or municipal legislature. A lobbyist ordinarily attempts to influence a legislator either by presenting the strongest case possible for his or her position on a particular bill that has been introduced or by encouraging the legislator to introduce a bill that in the lobbyist's view provides needed legislation. An example of the latter would be the lobbying done by many members of state speech-language-hearing associations to have licensure bills for professionals in our field introduced. A lobbyist may be a full- or part-time professional who is paid by a special interest group or he or she may be a volunteer. The approach that he or she uses may include one or more of the following:

- "Bribery."
- Writing letters or sending telegrams (or mailgrams).
- Engaging in face-to-face discussions to explain in detail the reasons for the position being advocated.
- Testifying before legislative committees.
- Preparing briefs, memorandums, legislative analyses, and draft legislation for use by legislative committees and individual legislators.

Each of these approaches is discussed elsewhere in this chapter.

Lobbyists are granted to right to attempt to influence legislators in the *First Amendment* to the U.S. Constitution:

> *Congress shall make no laws . . . abridging the freedom of speech, or of the press, or the right of the people peaceably to assemble,* and to petition the Government for a redress of grievances *[emphasis mine]*.

This right is based largely on the guarantees of free speech and the peoples' right "to petition the Government for a redress of grievances." Lobbyists have attempted to influence legislators on federal, state, and municipal levels since the founding of our country (Schriftgiesser, 1951; *The Washington Lobby*, 1971).

Ethical lobbyists (as opposed to unscrupulous ones) make a genuine contribution to the legislative process. Legislators are unlikely to be knowledgeable about the subject matter of all the bills on which they are expected to vote. To cast an informed vote on a bill, legislators must understand the implications of both its being passed and defeated. Lobbyists representing *special interest groups* that have different points of view about a particular bill can help legislators understand the implications of its being passed and defeated. (Individuals having strong points of view about particular bills can do the same thing—in fact, while doing so they are functioning as lobbyists.) Consequently, lobbyists provide legislators with information that is highly likely to enable them to create better laws than they probably would be able to otherwise. In a sense lobbyists advocating various positions on an issue perform a similar service for *legislators* that attorneys representing plaintiff and defendant do in a trial for a *judge and jury*—that is, presenting the strongest case they can for their side, thereby maximizing the probability that an appropriate decision will be reached.

Most organizations encourage lobbying for legislation that is directly or indirectly related to the special interest that is shared by their members. People join an organization presumably because it allows them to interact with others who share an interest: The organization, thereby, becomes a credible "spokesperson" for persons having that special interest. The organization, if it is a relatively large one, may retain professional lobbyists to monitor pending legislation and when appropriate, present its points of view to legislators. Or it may have some of its members perform these functions. Or it may rely on a combination of professional lobbyists and volunteer ones to do so. The American Speech-Language-Hearing Association uses the latter approach (*Congressional Action Contact Network Handbook*, 1991). The organization employs professional lobbyists to monitor pending legislation and present its point of view to legislators and members of their staffs. It also uses member volunteers (CAC Network) to present its points of view on pending legislation to members of Congress when the staff of its Governmental Affairs Department believes that doing so could be helpful.

An organization (such as ASHA) through its lobbying activities can *indirectly* promote the welfare of its members by promoting the welfare of those who are consumers of the goods and services that its members provide. If the American Speech-Language-Hearing Association, for example, supported legislation that would fund clinical services for a segment of the communicatively impaired population that is currently being underserved, it also would be creating additional employment opportunities for its members. Consequently, the motivation of an organization to lobby for the welfare of those who consume the goods and/or services that its members provide is partially altruistic and partially self-serving.

APPROACHES USED BY LOBBYISTS TO INFLUENCE LEGISLATORS

Lobbyists, as I indicated previously, have used a number of approaches (singly or in combination) to influence legislators' votes. Some implications of each of them are indicated in this section.

"Bribery"

Bribery is one of the oldest approaches that has been used to influence legislators. In its most blatant form, it involves the payment of money (or its equivalent) to legislators in exchange for their supporting or not supporting a particular bill. The ABSCAM scandal of the early 1980s in which an FBI agent posing as a lobbyist offered bribes to a number of members of Congress (which they accepted) for their support on a particular bill indicates that attempted bribery in its most blatant form can still occur. This approach does have a serious limitation other than being expensive; it's a *crime* for a lobbyist to offer a bribe and for a legislator to accept one.

The form of bribery in which a legislator is paid directly for a vote probably occurs relatively infrequently. There is, however, an indirect form of bribery practiced by special interest groups, that is not a crime and that appears to be quite widespread—that is, political action committees (PACs) making contributions to the *campaign funds* of certain persons who are running for election or reelection to a legislature (municipal, state, or federal). If they are elected, they may feel obligated to the special interest groups who supported them financially, which could influence their votes on certain legislation. ASHA, through its Political Action Committee (ASHA-PAC), contributes to the campaign funds of some of the persons who are running for election or reelection to Congress (ASHA-PAC: A visible influence, 1988; ASHA-PAC wants effective leaders, 1990; Koenigknecht, 1990).

There is another form of "bribery" used by lobbyists that ordinarily is not regarded as being such. An example would be a lobbyist arranging to have a legislator address the special interest group that he or she represents. The legislator probably would receive some media coverage for his or her presentation and an honorarium.

Writing Letters and Sending Telegrams

A letter or telegram from a constituents that cogently argues his or her point of view on a bill can influence how the legislator will vote on it. The likelihood that it will do so is, in part, a function of how it is written. It should be "personal—clearly handwritten or typed. Nothing looks worse to a legislator than an obvious, orchestrated campaign. There is no substitute for a carefully worded, thoughtful letter [or telegram] from a constituent" (*Congressional Action Contact Network Handbook*, 1991).

The following are some DOs and DON'Ts that ASHA recommends should be followed when corresponding with a legislator (*Congressional Action Contact Network Handbook*, 1991):

The Fundamental DOs

DO address . . . [the legislator] properly.

Proper form for addressing . . . members of Congress:

Honorable (full name)	Honorable (full name)
U.S. House of Representatives	U.S. Senate
Washington, DC 20515	Washington, DC 20510
Dear Representative:	Dear Senator:

DO write legibly. (Typed letters are preferable, but handwritten letters are acceptable if they are readable.)

DO use your own words and personal or business stationery.

DO be brief and to the point. Discuss only single issues or related issues in each letter.

DO identify your subject clearly; give the name of the legislation or the bill number if you know it.

DO state your reason for writing. Cite personal experiences and show how the issue would affect you, the professions, the population you serve, and the district the legislator represents.

DO draw attention to the personal connection you may have with the legislator or a time you met.

DO ask the legislator to state his or her position on the issue when replying to your letter. As a constituent you are entitled to know.

DO request specific action; tell the legislator what you want him or her to do.

DO be sure to include your address and sign your name legibly. If you have family, business, or political connections related to the issue, explain them. They may serve as identification when your point of view is considered.

DO feel free to write if you have a question or problem dealing with procedures of governmental departments. Congressional offices often can help you cut through red tape or give advice that can save you time and effort.

DO include pertinent editorials from local papers.

DO time your letters for maximum effect. Write early in a session when bills are introduced if you have ideas about an issue that you would like to see incorporated into legislation. If . . . [a legislator] is a member of a committee to which it has been referred, write when the committee begins hearings. If the legislator is not a member of the committee handling the bill, write just before the bill comes to the floor for debate and vote.

DO write the chairman, chairwoman, or members of the committee holding hearings on legislation that interests you, especially if you have facts that could influence his or her thinking.

DO write to say you approve, not just to complain or oppose. Public officials hear mostly from constituents who oppose their actions.

DO thank . . . [them] if they have taken a position or cast a vote that you think is right on a particular issue. Knowing that constituents approve of their actions is important to legislators and will help reaffirm the position when the issue comes up again.

The Fundamental DON'Ts

DON'T apologize for taking his or her time. If you are brief and to the point, he or she is glad to hear from you.

DON'T be argumentative; you are trying to convince the legislator to incorporate your views into his or her legislative positions.

DON'T be vague. Some letters received in congressional offices are couched in such general terms that they leave Senators/Representatives and their staffs wondering what the writer had in mind.

DON'T try to cover too many issues in a single letter . . . It is best to limit the content of your letter to one issue that is particularly pertinent to you. If there are several unrelated issues (e.g., preschool education and biomedical research), it is best to cover them in separate letters. Chances are these issues will be handled by different staff in the congressional office.

DON'T write to your legislator's local district office unless your correspondence deals with a local issue. You will receive a quicker response when you use the Washington, DC address. . . .

Face-to-Face Discussions with Legislators

Meeting a legislator personally can be an effective method for communicating your point of view on a bill. The likelihood that your get-together will influence the legislator in the way you desire is, in part, a function of how you conduct yourself prior to and during the session. The following *DOs* and *DON'Ts* for a successful meeting have been suggested by ASHA (*Congressional Action Contact Network Handbook*, 1991):

DOs

DO make an appointment in advance; you will be scheduled for a specific amount of time, and you will be asked what the subject matter is. Be sure to stick to the scheduled amount of time allotted you.

DO be on time for your scheduled appointment. Be prepared to wait.

DO be flexible. If the member cannot meet with you at the scheduled time, reschedule an appointment or meet with the Administrative or Legislative Assistant.

DO be prepared. Present pertinent facts, figures, opinions. Be brief, articulate, and persuasive; get to the point; have material to back up your position.

DO give the legislator a chance to talk; you may be surprised at his or her knowledge and/or questions.

DO keep on the subject of discussion; do not let the conversation stray to other subjects.

DO leave materials that repeat your major points with the staff.

DO get to know the legislator's staff, especially the administrative and/or legislative assistant. Because of the volume and complexity of legislation, Members of Congress rely on their staffs to do research, watch the progress of legislation of interest to constituents, and prepare summaries and recommendations on the various measures. The better informed the aide is, the more complete his or her recommendations can be for the legislator.

DO follow up your meeting with a letter of thanks; include a summary of the points you made at the meeting.

DO use the proper salutation when meeting with . . . [the legislator] (Senator ____ or Congressman/Congresswoman or Representative ____.)

DON'Ts

DON'T make the meeting too long; offer to send any additional information that may have been requested by mail.

DON'T give up on the Member because he or she doesn't vote your way on every issue. You don't know what his or her commitments are on many issues. Give him or her the benefit of the doubt.

DON'T argue if the Member doesn't give you a definite positive position. Keep the lines of communication open; if the Member is not on your side today, he or she may be two months from now.

DON'T overlook the staff aides in the office. They can be very influential with the legislator.

Meetings with members of Congress can be set up at their local district offices when the body is in recess. While it is in session they can be scheduled at their office in Washington, DC.

Testifying before Legislative Committees

Before a bill is considered by a particular legislative body (such as the Senate or House of Representatives), it ordinarily is considered by a *committee* made up of members of that body. The mandate given to this committee is to conduct a *hearing* to explore the ramifications of the bill thoroughly. Following the hearing, the committee is expected to recommend what action the legislative body should take on the bill. Lobbyists and others representing special interest groups ordinarily are permitted to testify at these hearings. Their testimony consists of arguments, supported by evidence, indicating why they believe (or the group they represent believes) that the bill under consideration should or should not be enacted into law. Those who testify usually are questioned by members of the committee following their formal presentation. (To learn more about the nature of such testimony, watch a House or Senate hearing for several hours on one of the C-SPAN cable television channels.) Officers of the American Speech-Language-Hearing Association and members of its Governmental Affairs Department staff have testified at such hearings. Officers of state associations and lobbyists retained by them have testified at similar hearings conducted by state legislative committees.

Preparing Briefs, Memorandums, Legislative Analyses, and Draft Legislation

Lobbyists often draft documents for individual legislators and legislative committees. Such a document may contain statistical or other data that support a position that the lobbyist is advocating. Or it may summarize the organization's position on certain pending legislation. Or it may be a preliminary draft of a bill. A state speech-language-hearing association that wanted a licensure bill passed by its state legislature might prepare a preliminary draft of such a bill and then have its lobbyist attempt to locate one or more legislators who would be willing to sponsor it.

FUNCTIONING AS A LOBBYIST

Many speech-language pathologists and audiologists would be at least a little unnerved by the thought of contacting one of their state or federal legislators and attempting to influence his or her vote on a bill. They tend to regard their state and federal legislators as authority figures who deal mainly with issues that affect the majority of their constituents, and consequently, are unlikely to have much interest in the problems of persons who are handicapped. This is *not* their attitude toward them. If it were, the Americans with Disabilities Act of 1990, for example, would never have been passed.

Lobbyists function as *behavior modifiers*. They attempt to *shape* the behavior of legislators. Their overall behavioral objective is to get legislators sponsor a particular bill or vote in a particular way on it. To achieve their objective, they consciously or unconsciously use principles of behavior modification. They present arguments supported by data to legislators who are not sympathetic to their points of view and then *positively reinforce* any comments the legislators make that suggest their attitudes are changing.

What are a lobbyist's objectives? The main one is to convince legislators that the positions he or she is advocating are valid and consequently, they should "do the right thing" by voting in a particular way or by sponsoring a particular bill. And furthermore, to convince them that they are likely to benefit from doing so. Even if legislators are convinced that a particular position is valid, they may not support it if they believe that doing so could hurt their chances for reelection.

For further practical information about lobbying, see the *Congressional Action Contact Network Handbook* (1991), Browne (1991), and Wolpe (1990).

PLAYING AN ADVOCACY ROLE

Our focus in this chapter thus far has been on supporting the passage of bills that benefit persons who are communicatively impaired. After such a bill has been passed, we may have an opportunity to serve as an *advocate* for persons who could benefit from it. In this role we would do everything possible to insure that our clients receive the services they are entitled to under the law. A client may not receive services to which he or she is legally entitled unless his or her clinician is willing to assume this responsibility.

Why might communicatively impaired persons not receive services to which they are legally entitled? There could be several reasons. One is that they are not aware of the existence of governmental programs from which they could obtain the necessary funding. For example, in Wisconsin there was a program when this chapter was written that funded telecommunication devices for its citizens who were deaf, hard of hearing, or severely speech impaired of which many who could benefit were unaware.

A second reason why persons who are entitled by law to receive certain services do not receive them is that the responsible agency is unwilling to provide them. A state department of public instruction, for example, could refuse to fund clinical services for middle-school-age children whose only articulation error is a substitution of w/r, even though it can be argued that under federal law (P.L. 94-142) they are entitled to receive such services.

The ethical responsibility mentioned elsewhere in this chapter to "hold paramount the welfare of persons served professionally" refers to advocacy as well as to lobbying. Holding paramount the welfare of clients implies doing whatever one can to make it possible for them to receive the clinical services they require. Consequently, it implies an obligation to play an advocacy role.

How can you satisfy your ethical obligation to be an advocate for persons who are communicatively impaired? The answer to this question depends on why a client may not be receiving needed services. If a client (or his or her family) is unaware of programs and organizations from which funding may be available, you could provide him or her with information about them (see Tucker & Goldstein, 1991). Of course, to be able to do this you would have to stay current with regard to municipal, state, and federal programs—as well as those of nongovernmental (e.g., service) organizations—that could provide such funding.

You may also be able to play an advocacy role by attempting to convince program administrators to fund services that they are not currently funding. Most medical insurance programs during the 1970s did not fund electronic augmentative communication aids. Some speech-language pathologists played an advocacy role by arguing that such aids are a type of *prosthesis* (i.e., a communication prosthesis) and were, therefore, fundable under existing regulations.

Another way that you may be able to play an advocacy role is by providing advice to clients and their families that could assist them in obtaining services that they are being denied, in spite of the fact that they are entitled to them by law. What advice might you give them that could facilitate their obtaining such services? Perhaps the best advice you could give would be to *threaten legal action* (i.e., a civil suit) if the services or funds are not provided. Most government agencies will go to great lengths to avoid such litigation, particularly if they know they will probably lose. It can be very costly to an agency to lose such litigation because if a court decides that they have to provide services they are not currently providing, it would establish a precedent that would be likely to result in requests from others for the services. Consequently, an agency so threatened is likely to find a way to "quietly" provide the services rather than risk litigation.

REFERENCES

ASHA-PAC: A visible influence. (1988). *Asha*, 30 (9), 57.

ASHA-PAC wants effective leaders. (1990). *Asha*, 32 (8), 33.

Browne, J. T. (1991). May you live with "interesting" laws: Government regulation in the 1990s. *Asha*, 33 (6), 39–40.

Congressional Action Contact Network Handbook (1991). Rockville, MD: American Speech-Language-Hearing Association.

Koenigsknecht, R. A. (1990). Go in the name of the law. *Asha*, 32 (11), 7–8.

Schriftgiesser, K. (1951). *The Lobbyists*. Boston: Little, Brown.

Tucker, B. P., & Goldstein, B. A. (1991). *Legal Rights of Persons with Disabilities*. Horsham, PA: LRP Publications.

The Washington Lobby (1971). Washington, DC: Congressional Quarterly.

Wolpe, B. C. (1990). *Lobbying Congress: How the System Works*. Washington, DC: Congressional Quarterly.

▶ 7

Participating in Trials and Hearings

You may be asked to testify at least once during your professional career as either an ordinary or an expert witness at a civil or criminal court proceeding or at a hearing. Such a hearing could, for example, be conducted under the auspices of an administrative agency such as a state department of public instruction or a local school board to comply with certain requirements of Public Law 94-142.

An ordinary ("fact") witness "testifies to what he [or she] has seen, heard, or otherwise observed" (Black, 1968, p. 1178). An audiologist might be asked to testify about the hearing of a person whom he or she had tested. Or a speech-language pathologist might be asked to testify about the therapy that he or she had used with a client. Ordinary witnesses testify about events that they have observed—their role ordinarily is to provide rather than evaluate evidence. Their only special qualifications are that they were present when an event occurred and are willing and able to describe what they observed.

Expert witnesses, on the other hand, both provide and evaluate evidence. Their special qualifications are that they possess "particular knowledge, wisdom, skill, or information regarding subject matter under consideration, acquired by study, investigation, observation, practice or experience and not likely to be possessed by the ordinary layman or inexperienced person" (Black, 1968, p. 688) and that they have "acquired ability to deduce correct inferences from hypothetical stated facts, or from facts involving scientific or technical knowledge" (Black, 1968, p. 688).

They can assist the judge, the jury, and the attorney who retains them in performing their functions, particularly with regard to dealing with subject matter that requires more than a layperson's knowledge to evaluate and/or comprehend.

Expert witnesses may or may not testify in a court or at a hearing. If they do not do so, they may testify in a *deposition* (testimony given under oath with attorneys for both parties present) prior to the trial or hearing or they may merely function as consultants to the attorneys who retain them. An expert witness's remarks, conclusions, and opinions ordinarily are protected when he or she is functioning as a consultant—they do not have to be communicated to the opposing attorney. Of course, the attorney who retains the expert may do so if he or she feels that communicating it is likely to help his or her client (e.g., encourage the other party to either drop the suit or accept an out-of-court settlement).

When expert witnesses give depositions and/or testify in court or at a hearing, their remarks, conclusions, and opinions ordinarily are not protected and will be painstakingly scrutinized by the opposing attorney. The opposition will attempt—through the process of cross-examination—to reduce the positive impact of their testimony on the judge and jury by casting doubt on their credibility as experts and/or the validity of their conclusions and opinions. The attorney who retains the expert witness will attempt to establish the expert's credibility and the validity of his or her testimony sufficiently strongly so that even after cross-examination the testimony will have the desired impact on the judge and jury.

ISSUES ABOUT WHICH SPEECH-LANGUAGE PATHOLOGISTS AND AUDIOLOGISTS HAVE TESTIFIED AS EXPERT WITNESSES

Expert witnesses function in both civil and criminal court proceedings and in hearings. Speech-language pathologists and audiologists have testified as experts in all three types of proceedings. Some of the issues about which they have testified are indicated in this section.

Criminal Court Proceedings

Speech-language pathologists and audiologists have probably been asked most often to provide expert testimony in criminal cases to either establish the competency of a defendant to be tried or to confirm the identification of a defendant.

Under our legal system, a person ordinarily cannot be tried and convicted for committing a crime unless he or she is judged legally competent. An aspect of being legally competent is being able to comprehend what is transpiring during one's trial. "In the United States of America it is a firmly established principle of law that a person cannot be put on trial if his [or her] condition is such that he [or she] will not be able to understand the proceedings and make a proper defense" (Meyers, 1968, p. 130). This ordinarily would be the case for someone who is deaf and neither able to speak nor understand speech or American Sign Language. It would also likely be the case for someone who has severe receptive or global aphasia. An expert witness in such instances would assess the communicative competence of the defendant and express an opinion about it in a deposition and/or in court.

The prosecution in some criminal cases has introduced as evidence an identification of a defendant based on the person's speech, voice, or fluency (e.g., whether he or she is a stutterer—see Bloodstein, 1988 and Shirkey, 1987). The identification of persons from their speech, voice, or fluency patterns is controversial, and speech-language pathologists have been asked to testify as expert witnesses both supporting (for the prosecution) and questioning (for the defense) the validity and reliability of such identifications.

Civil Court Proceedings

Speech-language pathologists and audiologists have been asked to provide expert testimony in competency hearings, personal injury cases, and divorce cases involving the custody of minors.

Communicative disorder specialists have been asked to testify about a person's competence to continue to manage his or her financial and other affairs. Some members of an aphasic's family, for example, may seek to have him or her declared incompetent to do so (Rada, Porch, & Kellner, 1975). A speech-language pathologist in this type of litigation could testify as an expert for either the family or the aphasic.

In personal injury cases the court must establish the extent of the injury and the prognosis for improvement before it can determine how much compensation the injured party should be awarded. Such cases include proceedings for malpractice (see Chapter 5) and worker's compensation. A speech-language pathologist or audiologist may be asked to evaluate someone's speech, language, and/or hearing and render an opinion about the extent to which the person's communicative disorder is handicapping to him or her. An audiologist, for example, may be asked to testify as an expert about the hearing of a person who is seeking worker's compensation for a hearing loss that she claims resulted from exposure to high levels of noise at her place of employment. Or a speech-language pathologist may be asked to testify as an expert about the aphonia of a person who is suing an anesthetist for malpractice because he claims that the anesthetist damaged his vocal folds when he passed a tube between them during a surgical procedure.

A speech-language pathologist or audiologist may be asked to testify as an expert in divorce litigation pertaining to the custody of minor children. Family courts are supposed to award the custody of minor children to the parent who can best meet their needs. In custody cases speech-language pathologists and audiologists ordinarily testify about such matters as the therapy and special educational needs of the child and the likelihood of these needs being met where each parent plans to reside. They might also testify about the ability of each parent to cope with problems arising from the child's communicative disorder. One parent, for example, may be able to understand almost all of a dysarthric child's speech and the other very little of it.

Administrative Agency Hearings

Administrative agencies conduct hearings that are somewhat similar in format to court proceedings. In fact, they are sometimes referred to as quasi-judicial proceedings. One feature they share with court proceedings is the use of expert witnesses. A speech-language pathologist or audiologist is probably more likely to be asked to testify as an expert at such a hearing than he or she is at a civil or criminal court proceeding.

Speech-language pathologists and audiologists have testified frequently as experts at hearings related to the enforcement of Public Law 94-142, which mandates local school districts to meet the special educational needs of all children who reside in the geographical area(s) that they serve. If the parents of a child feel that their school district is not adequately meeting his or her needs, they can request a hearing at which they are likely to be represented by an attorney. If the child has a communicative disorder and the parents question the appropriateness of the intervention the school district is providing, their attorney may ask a speech-language pathologist or audiologist to examine the child and testify as an expert about the child's special educational needs and the services required. Or the attorney representing the school district may make such a request in an attempt to establish that it is adequately meeting the child's needs.

SERVING AS AN EXPERT WITNESS

How should you conduct yourself while serving as an expert witness in a hearing or court proceeding? Some guidelines are presented in this section that were synthesized from several sources that endeavor to prepare physicians to serve as expert witnesses. The order in which topics are discussed does not necessarily indicate their importance. These guidelines are intended to supplement rather than substitute for a pretrial (or prehearing) conference with the attorney for whose client(s) you are testifying.

Projecting an Appropriate Image

The impact that an expert's testimony has on a judge and jury is determined not only by what the expert says, but also by how the expert conducts himself or herself while testifying. If the judge and jury perceive the expert as someone who is not highly confident about the accuracy of his or her testimony, they will tend to give the testimony less weight than they would otherwise. Furthermore, if the expert does not dress appropriately (i.e., in a manner consistent with expectations about how an "expert" should dress) or communicate well, his or her testimony may be given less credibility than it deserves. While it is unfortunate that the manner in which expert witnesses conduct themselves can profoundly influence the impact of their testimony on a judge and jury, it is nevertheless a fact of life with which they must contend. Consequently, it is crucial that persons testifying as experts conduct themselves in a manner that maximizes the likelihood that a judge and jury will give appropriate weight to their testimony.

A number of variables can influence the image that an expert witness projects, including the following:

- The amount of eye contact the expert has with the judge and jury (particularly the latter). Having frequent eye contact with them while testifying ordinarily will enhance a witness's image.

- The extent to which the expert can maintain his or her composure. The more successful the expert witness is at reflecting confidence and assurance while testifying, the more credence the judge and jury are likely to give to the testimony. Consequently, during cross-examination the opposing attorney is likely to attempt to get the expert to "lose it."
- The extent to which the witness establishes his or her qualifications to testify as an expert on the matter at hand. The more successful he or she is in doing so, the more impact the testimony is likely to have on the judge and jury. The opposing attorney is likely to attempt to reduce the impact of his or her testimony by questioning the witness's qualifications as an expert on the subject.
- The extent to which the witness succeeds at communicating with the judge and jury. Some experts attempt to impress a jury by using many esoteric scientific terms. This is a questionable strategy. A jury is more likely to be persuaded by an expert who attempts to communicate with them in language that they can understand. An expert witness should assume that the members of the jury know nothing about his or her field of expertise and take on a responsibility to communicate findings and opinions to them in language they can understand. Obviously, while doing this he or she should be careful not to appear to be talking down to them.
- The extent to which the expert has reviewed the testimony with the attorney who retained him or her. If the attorney either is unaware of or does not understand what the expert can say that may be helpful to the client, the attorney may not ask the appropriate questions during direct examination. An expert witness ordinarily testifies during direct examination by answering a series of questions asked by the attorney who retained him or her. If all of the questions that need to be answered in order to present the testimony are not asked, then the expert's testimony may not have the desired impact on the judge and jury. The attorney may ask the expert to formulate a series of questions, the answers to which will enable the expert to communicate his or her opinion(s) in a relatively complete, clear, and organized manner.

A second reason why the expert should review the testimony with the attorney who retained him or her is to alert the attorney to how the testimony is likely to be attacked during cross-examination. If the attorney is aware of how it is likely to be attacked, he or she can be better prepared to "repair the damage" during redirect examination.

- The directness with which the expert answers questions. If the expert is perceived by the judge and jury as being evasive or defensive when answering questions, the potential positive impact of the testimony on them is likely to be reduced. An expert witness must be particularly careful not to appear evasive when asked by the opposing attorney (during cross-examination) to answer "yes" or "no" to a question that the expert believes cannot be adequately answered with a simple "yes" or "no." In such a situation an expert witness is permitted to appeal to the judge. The judge may allow the witness to give a fuller answer, but if not, the expert should not argue about it. The attorney who retained the expert can provide him or her an opportunity to answer more fully during the redirect examination.
- The respect the expert shows for the judge and jury. The judge is the "boss" of the court and the expert witness should always show respect. Failure to do so can adversely affect the image that the members of the jury have of the expert since they tend to expect witnesses to be respectful of the judge. It can also result in the expert being held in contempt of court.
- Whether the jury believes the expert is being paid for testifying. An expert witness ordinarily receives a fee—not for the testimony, but for his or her time, professional knowledge, and services for studying the facts of the case and rendering opinions based on them. If the opposing attorney (during cross-examination) can make the jury believe that the expert testified as he or she did because of the fee received, they are apt to give little weight to the testimony.

Testifying

An expert witness's testimony can ordinarily be divided into four parts. The first consists of answers to questions about personal background and experience that are asked by the attorney who retained him or her. Its purpose is to establish credibility to testify as an expert about the matter at hand.

The second part consists of answers to questions about the case, which are asked by the attorney who retained him or her. These questions and answers are the "meat" of the expert's direct testimony.

The third part consists of answers to questions about the direct testimony, which are asked by the opposing attorney. These questions are likely to deal both with the expert's qualifications to testify as an expert about the matter at hand and with the expert's testimony about the case. This part is referred to as cross-examination. It is an attempt to nullify the expert's direct testimony by suggesting to the jury that he or she is not qualified to testify as an expert about the matter at hand and/or that his or her interpretations (opinions) are not the only possible ones.

The fourth part consists of answers to questions about the expert's testimony during cross-examination that are asked by the attorney who retained him or her. The attorney's objective during this part (which is referred to as the redirect examination) is to reestablish the qualifications of the witness and to establish that the interpretations (opinions) given in testimony are more viable than those suggested by the opposing attorney during cross-examination.

Some guidelines for your testifying as an expert during each of these four parts are presented in the following paragraphs.

Being Qualified as an Expert

The first task of the attorney who retained you is to establish during direct examination that you are competent to testify as an expert about the matter at hand. If the attorney is successful, the trial judge will rule that you are competent to do so. The attorney will then go on to the substantive part of the direct examination.

To qualify you as an expert, the attorney will ask you a series of questions. The following series is representative:

Will you state your name, please?

Will you state your business address, please?

What is your business occupation?

What is your present title?

For how long have you been employed in this occupation?

Will you briefly describe, please, the subject matter of this occupation?

Do you specialize within this occupation?

What is your specialty?

What is it concerned with?

How long have you been in practice in this specialty?

What is your formal education?

What undergraduate school did you attend?

What degree did you obtain there?

What was your major field of study?

What graduate school(s) did you attend?

What degree(s) did you obtain there?

What was your major field of study?

What postgraduate training have you received?

Are you licensed (or certified) to practice this occupation?

By whom was this license (or certification) awarded?

For how long have you had it?

What positions have you held since the completion of your formal training?

For how long did you hold each?

To what professional organizations do you belong?

What are the qualifications for becoming a member of these organizations?

What offices and committee assignments have you held in these organizations?

Have you taught courses in your specialty?

Where?

Have you published articles or books?

How many articles have you published?

In what scientific journals did they appear?

How many books have you published?

What are the titles of your books?

What topics did you discuss in your articles and books?

Have you ever testified in court as an expert witness?

What subjects have you testified on?

How many clients diagnosed as having _____ have you treated?

Have you ever previously evaluated a client for (e.g., competency to manage his financial affairs)?

How many times have you performed such an evaluation?

The specific questions that you will be asked depend on your background and experience and the subject matter about which you will be testifying. If, for example, you have not published any articles or books, question pertaining to publication will not be asked.

The opposing attorney is entitled to cross-examine you about your qualifications. He or she may do so at this stage or wait until the direct examination has been completed.

You should not feel compelled to answer questions immediately after they are asked; it is wise to avoid appearing either too willing or reluctant. When answering, you should be brief and to the point, not volunteering extra information but answering only the questions asked. If a question is not clearly phrased, you should not hesitate to ask the attorney to clarify it. If the attorney makes an inaccurate remark or interprets testimony in a way that is not completely accurate, you should make a correction in a confident, but respectful, manner.

Direct Examination
After the trial judge rules that you are competent to testify as an expert, the attorney begins the questioning about the matter that is to be the subject of your testimony. Some questions are likely to be fact questions about the person who has the communicative disorder and the services the person has received. Others will be opinion questions. You may be asked to give an opinion based on the facts (evidence) in the case or a series of assumptions. The latter involves answering a hypothetical question. Your answer to such a question should conform to the facts that are substantiated in the evidence of the case.

You should avoid bringing written records to court if at all possible. When records are used while testifying, they become part of the evidence. The opposing attorney can examine them, comment on them, and read from them to the judge and jury. You would be unwise, therefore, to bring any written records that you would not want read aloud in court.

You will probably be allowed to use exhibits and demonstrations to clarify points that might otherwise be confusing to a jury. Exhibits can vary from anatomical diagrams (e.g., of the ear) to audiotapes or videotapes (e.g., to demonstrate the magnitude of the person's communicative disorder). Juries tend to be fascinated by demonstrations and exhibits that show the functions of the human body. You may request a blackboard if writing or drawing on it will help make certain points. While presenting exhibits and demonstrations, you should face the jury and address the members of it directly.

Cross-Examination

The opposing attorney is given the opportunity to cross-examine you after the direct examination has been completed. He or she will attempt to reduce or nullify any positive impact that your testimony has had on the jury. There are several strategies that may be used for this purpose. One is to attempt to raise questions in the minds of the jury members about your qualifications to testify as an expert on the matter at hand. If, for example, your testimony dealt with aphasia, the opposing attorney may attempt to show that your previous experience with aphasics has been quite limited and consequently, the correctness of your opinions is uncertain. Merely raising questions in the minds of the jury about the correctness of one aspect of your testimony can significantly reduce or nullify the impact of your testimony on them.

Another strategy that the opposing attorney may use to reduce or nullify to positive impact of your testimony is to raise questions in the minds of the jury about whether you were paid to testify in the way you did. The attorney would ask you if you were paid a fee for testifying. If you answer "yes," the attorney will attempt to use this to case doubt on the impartiality of your testimony. (This point is discussed in greater depth elsewhere in this chapter.) The attorney may also attempt to cast doubt on your impartiality by asking how many times you have testified as an expert. If the answer indicates a relatively large number of times, the attorney is likely to try to convince the jury that you are a "gun for hire."

A third strategy an opposing attorney may use of reduce or nullify the positive impact of your testimony is to convince the members of the jury that your opinions are not the only possible viable ones. The attorney could attempt to do this in several ways. He or she might attempt to get you to admit that your interpretations and opinions are not the only ones that would be consistent with the evidence. Or he or she may attempt to get you to say that you can't be completely certain about the accuracy of your testimony. Furthermore, he or she may introduce into evidence the testimony of his or her own expert witnesses that contradicts your testimony. By so doing, the attorney will attempt to convey the message to the members of the jury that experts disagree. Such a message, obviously, would tend to reduce the positive impact of your testimony.

You and the opposing attorney are adversaries during cross-examination. The attorney has a single objective—to induce you to behave (verbally and/or nonverbally) in a manner that will reduce or eliminate any positive impact that your testimony has had on the members of the jury. And you also should have a single objective—to project to the members of the jury an "image" that will not reduce any positive impact that your testimony has had on them and will possibly enhance it.

During cross-examination, the opposing attorney may attempt to reduce the positive impact of your testimony on the jury in one or more of the following ways:

- Cause you to become angry and counterattack. If the attorney is successful, the members of the jury are likely to perceive you as being less dignified than they originally thought, which could reduce the weight that they give your testimony.
- Cause you to lower your guard by behaving in a friendly manner. The opposing attorney behaves in a way that you interpret as relaxed and friendly. This is designed to cause you to lower your defenses and say things that will weaken your testimony. When the opposing attorney comes on in this way, you should raise rather than lower your guard.
- Intimidate you. A cross-examiner might grimly shuffle a batch of papers while approaching the witness stand to frighten you into thinking that they contain evidence damaging to your testimony. Or the cross-examiner might write down some of your responses in a very conspicuous manner, thereby suggesting that ammunition to destroy your testimony is being collected. If the attorney is successful and you exhibit overt signs of fright, not only might your credibility with the jury be reduced, but you may say things (because of not thinking clearly) that weaken your testimony.
- Cause you to agree that an opinion may be a speculation. If you agree with a cross-examiner that a particular opinion may be a speculation, the members of the jury may interpret this response to mean the opinion is mere guess-work. If a cross-examiner suggests that an opinion is speculation, you should indicate that it is not speculation, but is based on "reasonable professional certainty and in accordance with scientific probability" (Sanbar, 1977).
- Cause you to disparage the expert testimony for the opposite side. To do so could cause some members of the jury to lose respect for you, which could result in their giving your testimony less weight than

they would have given it otherwise. If during cross-examination you are asked to explain the conflicting expert testimony for the opposite side, you can answer by saying, "I am sure _____ is a competent professional, but I simply do not agree on this particular issue" (Sanbar, 1977).

- Cause you to answer a question with a "yes" that should be answered with a "no." A cross-examiner may ask you a series of questions at a relatively rapid rate, all of which call for the answer "yes" and then ask one that should be answered "no." Because of the rhythm you have developed to say "yes," you may end up saying "yes" when meaning to say "no."

Your testimony in some instances will end following cross-examination. If this is the case, the judge will indicate it. You should not leave the witness stand before being told to do so by the judge. It is important to maintain dignity when leaving the witness stand—never make any obvious victory signs or signs of relief, and do not grin broadly as a sign of triumph, or run away from the stand with unseemly haste (Sanbar, 1977).

Redirect Examination
The attorney who retained you may ask some additional questions to "repair the damage" that was done to your testimony during cross-examination. The points that you should keep in mind when answering such questions are the same as those mentioned in the section on direct examination.

THE EXPERT WITNESS FEE

An expert witness is ordinarily paid a fee to compensate for time and testimony-related expenses. He or she should seek to be paid an hourly rate rather than a lump sum fee. The hours that are compensated should include not only those spent in court (or at hearings) but also those incurred in making out reports, attending pretrial (or prehearing) conferences, and gathering data (including examining the person who has the communicative disorder). The expenses should include transportation costs, hotel rooms, meals, tips, time spent on the telephone, and consultations (Sanbar, 1977). He or she should carefully record and, if possible, document both the amount of time spent on a case and the expenses incurred.

It is unethical for an expert witness to enter into an agreement that makes the fee contingent on the outcome of the trial. However, it would not be unethical for him or her to agree to serve without guarantee of payment (Sanbar, 1977).

An expert witness should have a written agreement (contract) with the attorney who retains him or her to avoid misunderstandings. It should specify the amount to be paid, by whom, and when. This agreement should include a provision assuring compensation for preparations and services provided in the event of an out-of-court settlement. Most cases are settled out of court.

REFERENCES

Black, H. C. (1968). *Black's Law Dictionary* (Rev. 4th ed.). St. Paul, MN: West Publishing Company.

Bloodstein, O. (1988). Verification of stuttering in a suspected malingerer. *Journal of Fluency Disorders*, 13, 83–88.

Meyers, L. J. (1968). *The Law and the Deaf*. Washington, DC: Vocational Rehabilitation Administration.

Rada, R. T., Porch, B., & Kellner, R. (1975). Aphasia and expert medical witness. *American Academy of Psychiatry and the Law Bulletin*, 3, 231–237.

Sanbar, S. S. (May 1977). *The expert witness*. Paper presented at the American Academy of Private Practice in Speech Pathology and Audiology Conference on Legal Considerations, Oklahoma City.

Shirkey, E. A. (1987). Forensic verification of stuttering. *Journal of Fluency Disorders*, 12, 197–203.

▶ 8

Marketing Clinical Services

The marketing of clinical services has at least two things in common with report writing. Few clinicians yearn to do it and employers not only expect them to do it, but to do it well. To market clinical services successfully, you must acquire both an objective attitude toward doing it and information about how to do it. This chapter will hopefully facilitate your acquiring both the attitude and the information.

WHY IS IT NECESSARY TO MARKET CLINICAL SERVICES?

The Code of Ethics of the American Speech-Language-Hearing Association requires you to "hold paramount the welfare of persons served professionally." The persons whose welfare you are required to hold paramount are those who have communicative disorders. An aspect of holding their welfare paramount is enabling them to obtain the clinical services they need to manage their disorder. To do so, they have to be aware that the services exist and know where and how to obtain them. The role of marketing is to provide them with this information.

Are there persons with communicative disorders in the United States who are not benefiting from available services either because they do not know that they exist or where and how to obtain them? The answer to this question is yes. While there undoubtedly are persons who lack this information for all services, the numbers who lack it is larger for some than for others. For at least a few such services, the majority of persons who could benefit from them do not appear to be aware that they exist and/or where or how to get them.

An example when this chapter was written was telecommunication relay services (TRSs) for persons who are severely speech impaired. The Americans with Disabilities Act of 1990 required every state to establish a TRS to provide telephone services to its citizens who had a speech or hearing impairment that were "functionally equivalent" to those available to its other citizens (Silverman, 1998). When using a TRS, persons who are severely speech impaired keyboard messages to an operator, known as a communication assistant (CA), who voices them to those whom they call or who call them. They can hear what persons they call or who call them say through "hearing carryover." There is no charge for using a TRS—calls cost the same as they would ordinarily. The service is available 24 hours a day, 365 days a year, and there is no limit on the number of calls that can be made or on how long calls can last. Some states even partially or wholly fund text telephones and other augmentative communication devices that are needed to communicate with a TRS. While the exact number of severely speech impaired persons who are not using a TRS because of not being aware that they exist is unknown, there appears to be almost universal agreement among directors of state TRSs that the number is considerably more than 50 percent. As a consequence, many state TRSs when this chapter was written were investing a considerable portion of their marketing budgets to increasing the level of awareness of TRSs and how to use them in this population. They were doing this, in part, by attempting to increase the level of awareness of TRSs among speech-language pathologists. Their informal surveying suggested that many speech-language pathologists who treat persons who temporarily or permanently could benefit from using a TRS were not encouraging their clients to use a TRS because they were not knowledgeable about them. The TRSs were attempting, through marketing, to change this situation.

The lack of awareness of a clinical service may be local rather than national. In fact, it exists whenever a speech-language pathologist or audiologist offers a new service. Persons who can benefit from the service cannot do so unless they know that it exists. Failure to make an adequate effort to make persons who could benefit from a service aware of its existence can be viewed as a violation of the "spirit" of the ASHA ethical code because it is not consistent with "promoting the welfare of persons served professionally." The "tool" that we use for making persons who could benefit from a service aware of it is marketing.

HOW DOES MARKETING CLINICAL SERVICES DIFFER FROM MARKETING BREAKFAST CEREALS?

Marketing breakfast cereals and clinical services has a similar objective—*creating and maintaining a customer relationship.* However, the strategies used for marketing the two tend to be different because what the marketer has to accomplish is different. With breakfast cereals, the marketer must create a need for the product and convince potential consumers that the product is better than alternatives—other breakfast cereals as well as other things that they could eat for breakfast. With clinical services, on the other hand, the marketer does not have to create a need for the "product" or convince potential consumers that it is better than alternatives. His or her goal is merely to make potential consumers of a service aware that it exists and provide them with information about the service, including how to access it.

HOW HAVE CLINICAL SERVICES BEEN MARKETED?

A number of strategies have been used for informing persons who have a communicative disorder and their families about services from which they may be able to derive some benefit, including the following:

- A listing in the Yellow Pages of the telephone book. This is one of the oldest strategies that speech-language pathologists and audiologists have used for alerting consumers to their services. Some such listings include information about the services provided.
- Business cards. You give business cards to the persons you meet who are potential referrers. At least some of them are likely to consult their business card collection (which they may have scanned into a computer database) when making referrals.

- Inservice presentations to professional groups who are potential referral sources. Such groups include physicians and classroom teachers. Information is presented that will enable them to identify persons who may have a communicative disorder and consequently, may benefit from being treated by a speech-language pathologist or audiologist. It is hoped that this information will both enable and motivate them make a referral when they come upon such a person.
- Articles in newsletters and journals of professional groups who are potential referral sources. The content of such articles is essentially the same as that of the inservice presentations.
- Exhibits at the conventions of professional groups who are potential referral sources. The same types of information are presented at an exhibit booth though handouts and conversation that are presented in inservice presentations and the newsletter or journal articles.
- Open houses at clinical facilities for members of professional groups who are potential referral sources. These usually include a tour of the facility and informal conversations with staff members about the services offered.
- Talks to the general public about communicative disorders and the treatments available for them. These usually occur at the meeting of an organization, such as a PTO or other service organization. The program chairpersons of most nonprofessional organizations are constantly searching for professionals who will speak to their group for free or a small honorarium. Several members of the audience may have family or friends (now or in the future) who could be helped by a speech-language pathologist or audiologist.
- Articles in newspapers and magazines about communicative disorders and the treatments available for them. The information presented would be the same as that in talks to the general public. Since the author's affiliation would be indicated in the article, such an article would not only help to increase the awareness of the general public of communicative disorders and their treatments, but it would also increase their awareness of the author's facility and consequently, could result in referrals.
- Talks about communicative disorders and the treatments available for them on local radio call-in type talk shows. Such talks should increase the awareness of the general public of communicative disor-

ders and their treatments as well as the programs offered by your facility.

- Exhibits at local health fairs. These, like participations in radio talk shows, increase the awareness of the general public of communicative disorders and their treatments as well as the programs offered by your facility.
- Reports in local media about specific programs offered by your facility. Local media are particularly likely to be willing to do a report on new programs or those that are unique in some way.
- Articles describing programs offered by your facility for persons having a particular type of impairment in newsletters of local support organizations (e.g., the American Cancer Society).
- Inclusion in community health-care referral databases. Such computer databases already exist in some communities and many more are likely to have them in the near future.
- Follow-up letters and reports to referral sources. In addition to keeping them informed about what is being done for the children and adults whom they have referred, such letters and reports are likely to yield new referrals if they suggest to the referrer that the persons are being treated competently.
- Newsletters and announcements mailed to local referral sources. These describe the facility's clinical programs, particularly new and innovative ones. They also describe the activities and accomplishments of the facility's staff, including research, publications, and advanced training. The latter help to create an image of competence for the facility.
- Distributing calendars and other things (ballpoint pens) on which is printed the name of the facility. Care must the taken when selecting items to distribute in this way that the items create a conservative professional image rather than a commercial one for the facility.
- Community involvement. This helps to create a positive image for the facility in both the minds of the general public and potential referrers. An example of such involvement would be the facility's staff volunteering to be telephone answerers at a local TV telethon.

This list is not exhaustive. However, it does include the strategies that have been used most often to make people who could benefit from our services aware that they exist.

HOW CAN YOU CONTRIBUTE TO MARKETING SERVICES FOR PERSONS WHO ARE COMMUNICATIVELY IMPAIRED?

Our focus thus far has been on strategies that have been used for marketing clinical services. We will focus here on specific ways that speech-language pathologists and audiologists who are not primarily administrators can implement some of these strategies and by so doing, increase the likelihood (at least a little) that children and adults who can benefit from our services will receive them. These include the following:

- Inform people about the range of disorders that communicative disorders specialists treat whenever the opportunity presents itself. Many persons, including some health-care professionals, are not aware of the wide range of disorders that communicative disorders specialists treat. If you do this whenever the opportunity presents itself (and you will not bore people by doing so), it is likely that during your professional lifetime at least a few persons who would not have gotten help with their communicative disorder because of being unaware that help is available will receive the help that they require.
- Carry business cards at all times. Distributing them can yield both clients and referral sources.
- Inform referral sources about treatment decisions for persons whom they refer. Also, periodically inform referral sources about the progress of persons they referred whom you are treating, if your doing so is acceptable to them.
- Make certain that the reports you send to referral sources are well written and convey an image of competence. Reports that are vague and contain spelling and grammatical errors do not convey such an image. While it is certainly true that there isn't a one-to-one relationship between writing good reports and being a good clinician, few of the persons on whom you rely for referrals are probably going to have the opportunity to observe you doing therapy and consequently, they are going to base their judgment of your competence, at least in part, on your reports.
- Volunteer to do inservice presentations to potential referrers. In the schools these would include classroom teachers and administrators. And in medical settings these would include members of almost all health-care professions.

- Volunteer at least once every year or two to give a talk to the general public about communicative disorders. The group to which you give the talk could be a PTO, a service organization, a grange, a church group, and so on.
- Explore the possibility of your facility meeting one unmet need in your community for services for persons who have communicative disorders and/or their families. After you identify the need, prepare a proposal to submit to your supervisor in which you document the need, indicate how it can be met at your facility, and indicate the source(s) from which funding might be sought.

REFERENCES

Silverman, F. H. (1998). *The Telecommunication Relay Service Handbook*. Newport, RI: Aegis Publishing Group.

▶ 9

Coping with Managed Health Care

We are currently living in a society in which the majority of people are cost-conscious shoppers. They want quality at a price they can afford. They use coupons when shopping at the supermarket and delay purchasing clothing and other goods until they are on sale. They purchase items at resale shops and at rummage (garage, tag) and estate sales.

Their desire for quality at a price that they can afford has also affected their shopping for health care. Rather than paying for health-related services as they are needed, they are purchasing health-care/insurance plans that provide a wide range of health services for a fixed monthly fee. In most communities there is more than one such plan available. Consequently, to attract and retain purchasers a plan has to provide them with quality services at the lowest cost possible. One consequence of this stress on being cost effective is that the traditional patient-clinician relationship is replaced by a patient-manager-clinician one. These plans are referred to as managed care because they bring managers (MBA-types) into the patient-clinician (client-clinician) relationship.

This altering of the relationship between the patient and clinician is profoundly affecting the delivery of all health-care services, including those provided by speech-language pathologists and audiologists. Some of the changes that the managed health-care model has made in the practice of speech-language pathology and audiology are indicated in this chapter as well as strategies for coping with them that will enable us to continue to meet the requirement of the ASHA ethical code "to hold paramount the welfare of persons served professionally."

HOW DOES MANAGED HEALTH CARE DIFFER FROM TRADITIONAL FEE-FOR-SERVICE?

Traditionally, patients (or their insurance companies) have paid health-care workers for services when they receive them. This is referred to as the "fee-for-service" model. The fee is set by the health-care worker and/or his or her employer and is billed either to the patient or to his or her insurance company. The practitioner decides what services the patient requires and cost is not usually a primary consideration. There is an incentive is to focus on treatment rather than prevention since treatment generates more income than prevention. The patient usually is not restricted with regard to the practitioners that he or she can use. And a practitioner is not obligated to have his or her therapy outcomes evaluated by anyone nor to demonstrate that the manner in which he or she is treating a patient is likely to benefit him or her in the real world.

Managed health-care plans differ in a number of ways from fee-for-services plans. Perhaps the most significant way that they differ is that services are *prepaid*. Moneys collected from members and/or their employers are allocated in advance to the plan's health-care professionals who then provide the members with the services they require. The amount of money that a health-care professional receives is not determined by the amount of service that he or she provides. A health-care professional receives the same amount from the moneys paid for a particular member each month regardless of whether he or she provides any services to that member that month. With fee-for-services plans, on the other hand, the amount of money that a health-care professional receives from a patient each month is determined by the services that he or she provides that patient each month. Consequently, the financial incentive for managed health-care plans differs from that for fee-for-services plans. With managed health-care plans, the fewer the services provided, the greater the profit. And with fee-for-services plans, the greater the number of services provided, the greater the profit. Consequently, it is not particularly surprising that managed health-care plans emphasize health maintenance—that is, prevention—and fee-for-services plans emphasize treatment. Other ways that managed health-care plans differ from fee-for-service plans are described elsewhere in the chapter.

HOW DOES MEDICAL INSURANCE DIFFER FROM MANAGED HEALTH-CARE PLANS?

With both, persons enrolled and/or their employers pay a certain amount each month. They differ, however, with regard to how moneys are allocated to health-care workers. From medical insurance, health-care workers are paid on a fee-for-service basis. And from managed health-care plans, they receive a fixed monthly fee for each person for whom they are responsible. Consequently, the financial incentive for health-care workers is not the same for both. With medical insurance, the more treatment a patient receives, the more money the health-care worker earns. With managed health-care plans, on the other hand, the less treatment a patient receives, the more money the health-care worker earns. Other ways that these two methods of funding impact on health care are mentioned elsewhere in the chapter.

The financial incentives associated with medical insurance are actually more complex than what was indicated in the preceding paragraph. While a health-care worker's income increases as amount of treatment increases, the insurance program's resources decrease as amount of treatment increases. Consequently, an insurance program may refuse to fund certain treatments (possibly by labeling them "experimental") because of the effect that funding them would have on its "bottom line."

One of the arguments against managed health-care plans is that they tend to discourage the use of expensive treatments. Medical insurance programs do also for the same reason—their bottom line. Consequently, this argument against managed health-care plans is actually an argument against any plan in which the person who receives a health-related service does not pay for it himself or herself.

MANAGED HEALTH CARE AND THE HEALTH MAINTENANCE ORGANIZATION (HMO)

Managed health-care plans have existed in the United States since the founding of the Western Clinic in Tacoma, Washington in 1906. They didn't, however, begin attracting relatively large numbers of members until after World War II. The numbers of such plans had increased to the point by the last third of this century that the Congress was motivated to pass the Health Maintenance Organization Act in 1973 to regulate their activities. For at least the past 25 years, the term Health Maintenance Organization, or HMO, has been used as a generic label for all managed health-care plans. Several organizational structures are used by managed health-care plans, one of which is the staff-based HMO (described elsewhere in this chapter). Consequently, the term HMO can be used as a label for either a specific type of managed health-care plan (staff-based HMO) or any managed health-care plan. In this chapter, the term HMO when not preceded by the words "staff-based" designates any managed health-care plan.

CHARACTERISTICS COMMON TO ALL HMOs

HMOs are not all structured the same way. The four most common structures are described elsewhere in the chapter. While the way in which an HMO is structured affects how it functions, all HMOs share a number of characteristics, including the following:

- They are corporations. While some are nonprofit, most currently are not.
- They combine financing and delivery of health-care services.
- They are tightly or loosely structured group practices that offer a wide range of health-care services.
- Enrollees prepay at set intervals (e.g., monthly) the same amount of money, regardless of the amount of services that they receive. They may, however, be required to make a small co-payment for some services (e.g., prescriptions).
- Health-care providers agree to dispense services for less than their usual fees.
- Health-care providers agree to accept a *capitation* payment method for their services. They receive a fixed periodic payment for each enrollee for whom they are responsible, regardless of the amount of services that they provide.
- The number one objective of health-care providers (at least theoretically) is to provide the best health-care services that they can from the moneys they receive as capitation payments.

- Health-care providers negotiate a capitation fee contract with the HMO. If they accept a capitation fee that is too low, they will lose money. If they request a capitation fee that is higher than another bidder will accept, they are unlikely to receive the contract. ASHA has data on reasonable capitation fees for communicative disorders specialists. Capitation fee contracts are subject to periodic renegotiation.
- Health-care providers are expected to use personnel and services associated with the HMO whenever possible. An otolaryngologist, for example, would be expected to refer patients to an audiologist associated with the HMO for hearing testing (assuming, of course, that there was an audiologist associated with it).
- Primary physicians—internists and pediatricians—usually serve as "gatekeepers." Patients are referred by them to other health-care professionals.
- Considerable resources are devoted to health maintenance—that is, preventing health problems and treating those that can't be prevented at an early stage (when they tend to be less expensive to treat).
- The services utilized by a health-care providers are monitored and reviewed by the HMO's utilization reviewers. Because referrals for diagnostic tests and specialty evaluations have to be justified, fewer tend to be made. Theoretically, those tests and evaluations that are not ordered under a managed care plan that would be ordered under a fee-for-services one are not really necessary.
- Their quality control personnel monitor the "real-world" impacts of services on enrollees. Those treatments for which there is not good documentation that they significantly improve a person's ability to function are less likely to be approved than others.
- If two treatments or devices (e.g., hearing aids) tend to produce essentially the same outcome, the less expensive one is likely to approved for utilization.
- Paraprofessionals and family members are utilized whenever doing so does not significantly reduce the likelihood of a good outcome.

CHECKS ON THE SERVICES PROVIDED BY HMOs

Since the fewer services an HMO provides its enrollees the more money it can make, what would motivate an HMO to provide its enrollees with all of the services that they require? There are a number of reasons why HMOs would regard it as being in their best interest to do so, including the following:

- Competition. There is usually more than one HMO operating in a community. If the word gets out through the media or otherwise that an HMO is not providing its enrollees adequate services, there are likely to be fewer new enrollees and at least some of those currently enrolled are likely to switch to another HMO when they have the opportunity to do so. Furthermore, businesses that have contracted with them for health care for their employees are not likely to renew their contracts. Consequently, an HMO's enrollees must regard its services as being satisfactory if it is to stay in business.
- Government regulation. The federal government regulates the functioning of HMOs in a number of ways. It can exert tremendous pressure on an HMO (directly or indirectly) to provide enrollees with the services with which it has contracted to provide them. It is likely to do so because both the President and the Congress are strongly supportive of the managed health-care model and, consequently, want the general public to view it favorably. Stories in the media about shortcomings of HMOs detract from this image.
- The contract between the enrollee and the HMO. The relationship between an enrollee and an HMO is a contractual one (see Chapter 4). If an HMO fails to live up to its contractual obligations to one of its enrollees, he or she can ask a court to force it to do so and to pay the enrollee's legal fees. If an HMO fails to live up to its contractual obligations to a number of its enrollees, a *class action suit* can be initiated. It is likely that an attorney could be found to represent the enrollees on a contingency fee basis (e.g., for one-third of any compensatory and punitive damages that the court awards the plaintiffs).
- The media. Stories in the media about an HMO not meeting its contractual obligations tend to threaten its survival.
- Peer review by an HMO's staff and its professional association(s). Both have an interest in correcting any problems that could damage the reputation and/or survival of an HMO.

TYPES OF HMOs

There are a number of basic types of HMO structures, including the following: staff-based HMOs, individual practice associations (IPAs), preferred provider organizations (PPOs), group practice HMOs, and network HMOs. The *staff-based HMO* is the oldest. A staff-based HMO is a complete medical center. It provides its enrollees with most (if not all) of the outpatient health-care services that they require under one roof. Its full-time physicians and other health-care providers are salaried employees. It closely orchestrates health-care services that it cannot provide and consequently, must contract for them from others. It may utilize nurse-practitioners or physician's assistants to handle some of the routine care. Medical specialists are available if needed. Some specialists may be at the center only on a part-time basis. Such specialists may work part-time for other HMOs and/or have a private practice. A speech-language pathologist or audiologist may also be employed by a staff-based HMO on a part-time basis.

The *individual practice association* (IPA) is now more common than the staff-based HMO. It represents an attempt to combine the best features of the staff-based HMO with those of the fee-for-services delivery system. An IPA is essentially a prepaid health-care plan that is offered by an association of physicians who are in private practice. Enrollees can use any primary care physician and specialists who belong to the IPA. Physicians and other health-care providers are paid on a fee-for-services basis by the managing arm of the association, which may be a separate legal entity. If it is set up as a separate legal entity, it is likely to be designated as an HMO and the combination of the physicians' association and it as an IPA-HMO.

Preferred provider organizations (PPOs) operate like IPAs except that enrollees can be treated by physicians who are not members of the PPO. Consequently, they are "open-use systems." Enrollees have full coverage (except for small copayments) when they are treated by a physician who belongs to the PPO. However, if they see a physician who is not a member of the PPO, the PPO will pay a portion of the cost of the visit. The difference between the physician's regular fee and what is paid by the PPO is billed to the enrollee.

A *group-practice HMO* consists of a small group of physicians in private practice who decide to incorporate and charge patients a standard monthly fee. The group may contain both primary-care physicians and specialists or it may be organized around a single specialty (e.g., cardiac care). The group may hire an HMO-management firm to provide administrative services. These tend to be the most loosely organized of all HMOs.

The *network HMO* is an extension of the group-practice HMO. It consists of a number of group practices that are linked together by an HMO-management firm in a manner that enables enrollees to use any practitioner within the network. A group practice within a network can be a specialty one—for example, one consisting of speech-language pathologists and/or audiologists who are in full- or part-time private practice.

THE ROLE OF THE PATIENT IN MANAGED HEALTH CARE

One aspect of managed health care is that patients and their families are expected to assume more responsibility for managing their health care than they were previously. Hospital stays tend to be shorter and outpatient surgery is on the increase. The motivation for these changes and this shift in responsibility is almost completely financial.

The financial pressures that have resulted in patients and their families assuming greater responsibility for medical care have also increased their responsibility for the management of their own or their family member's communicative disorder. A speech-language pathologist may manage a client's communicative disorder by training a family member to provide the necessary therapy (rather than doing it himself or herself), serving as a consultant to and "supervisor" for the family member, and monitoring and documenting progress. In some cases, a client will make more progress if his or her communicative disorder is managed in this way than he or she would if the clinician assumed full (or almost full) responsibility for management. Consequently, utilization of the managed-care philosophy will not necessarily result in poorer outcomes. Whether it does so is in large part a function of the flexibility and ingenuity of the clinician. A clinician who continues to utilize traditional clinical management approaches—that is, play the game by the old rules—is more likely to have poorer outcomes than one who attempts to adapt to the "new realities" and play the game by the rules now required to win. This need for flexibility and ingenuity to survive is dealt with further elsewhere in the chapter.

ETHICAL IMPLICATIONS OF MANAGED HEALTH CARE

It would be a violation of the spirit of the ASHA ethical code to allow the financial restrictions imposed by the managed health philosophy to impede our ability to "hold paramount the welfare of persons served professionally." We have an ethical responsibility to find cost-effective ways to continue doing what we have been doing—that is, reducing the severity of our clients' communicative disorders. Doing so may, for example, require us to relegate some of the responsibility for dispensing therapy to paraprofessionals, volunteers, or family members.

COPING STRATEGIES FOR SPEECH-LANGUAGE PATHOLOGISTS AND AUDIOLOGISTS

Perhaps your important coping strategy as a speech-language pathologists or audiologist is to accept the fact that the managed-care philosophy is not a fad but is here to stay. The specific forms that it will take in the future may not be those of the present HMO, IPA, or PPO. However, the desire to limit the growth of the cost of health care to that of inflation and at the same time more effectively utilize the funding available to help people cope with their environment is likely to exist into the foreseeable future.

Coping successfully in a managed health-care environment will require you to do a number of things. Perhaps the most important is managing your clients' communicative disorders in ways that are likely to be regarded by potential referrers and payers as being both cost-effective and helpful. For them to be cost-effective, you may have to utilize paraprofessionals, volunteers, and/or family members for doing some routine tasks—those that don't require your level of training to do adequately. Such tasks could include providing routine drill-practice language/cognitive stimulation to brain-damaged clients under your supervision. Rather than the use of others threatening your job security, the opposite is likely to be true. Because you would be managing your clients' disorders more cost-effectively than otherwise, you would be doing what referrers and payers in a managed care environment reward and, consequently, your job security would tend to be enhanced.

Not only must your therapy programs be cost-effective for you to survive in a managed care environment, they must also be helpful to those receiving them. They must enable those receiving them to cope more effectively in the "real world." Therapy programs for which there is scientific documentation for such benefits are more likely to be funded than those for which such documentation does not exist. Those who advocate the managed-care philosophy claim that they can hold down costs without reducing quality by curtailing funding to therapy programs that have not been demonstrated scientifically to help people function significantly more effectively in their environments. Consequently, a person having a communicative disorder may not be enough to justify therapy in a managed-care environment. There may also have to be some solid evidence that the therapy program being recommended is likely to result in the person being able to function more effectively in his or her environment. Whether or not you are required to present such evidence to justify doing therapy at your facility, your making it available to referrers and payers is likely to be respected and to enhance your job security. The gathering of such evidence is dealt with in Chapter 11.

The focus on functional outcomes and the need for scientific data to demonstrate them is a commendable feature of the managed health-care philosophy. If certain of the goals that we seek to accomplish do not enable our clients to function better in the "real world" and/or the management programs that we use to accomplish such goals are unlikely to enable us to do so, then we shouldn't be surprised if our requests for funding to accomplish them are rejected. If we want most of our requests for funding to be approved, we will have to focus on goals that if accomplished will improve clients' abilities to function in their environments. Furthermore, we will have to make outcome data available to payers that indicate the management programs we plan to use for achieving these goals are likely to be effective.

One task that you will be required to do if you negotiate a contract with an HMO is to set a capitation rate—the monthly amount you will receive for each member of a group to whom you agree to provide certain services. It is usually difficult to arrive at an appropriate one the first time because it is difficult to predict the amount of services that you will have to provide. I would strongly recommend that if you have to do this you contact ASHA. They have data that should enable you to develop at least a "first approximation" of a capitation rate. I further recommend that your first such contract should be a relatively short-term one—between six months and a year. You can then negotiate for an adjusted capitation rate if your guess on the level of service you are required to provide is too low.

Many publications contain information that can help you cope with the managed-care philosophy. Those that are particularly relevant for our field include Ad Hoc Committee on Managed Care (1994); Butler (1996);

Carter, Spiller, and Mather (1995); Council of State Association Presidents (1996); Landrum, Schmidt, and McLean (1995); Rubins (1996); and Vekovius (1995).

REFERENCES

Ad Hoc Committee on Managed Care. (1994). *Managing Managed Care.* Rockville, MD: American Speech-Language-Hearing Association.

Butler, K. (Summer, 1996). Managed care: Emerging issues in clinical ethics. *Asha,* 38, 7.

Carter, M., Spiller, M., & Mather, D. (1995). *Capitation Rates and Managed Care Manual.* McLean, VA: American Academy of Audiology and Academy of Dispensing Audiologists.

Council of State Association Presidents. (1996). *State Reference Guide on Managed Care in Speech-Language Pathology and Audiology.* Rockville, MD: American Speech-Language-Hearing Association.

Landrum, P., Schmidt, N., & McLean, A. (1995). *Outcome-Oriented Rehabilitation.* Gaithersburg, MD: Aspen.

Rubins, A. (February 20, 1996). ASHA lobbies to expand managed care access. *ASHA Leader,* 1 (4), 1–2.

Vekovius, G. T. (September, 1995). Managed care 101: Introducing managed care into the curriculum. *Asha,* 37, 44–47.

▶ 10

Using Paraprofessionals Advantageously

The use of paraprofessionals in the fields of speech-language pathology and audiology is not a new phenomenon. They have been utilized, particularly in the schools, for more than twenty-five years. The first official recognition of them by ASHA was perhaps a set of guidelines adopted by the Legislative Council in 1969 for their responsibilities, training, and supervision (ASHA, 1970). By 1981, many school districts were employing them and twenty four states had provisions for them in their speech-language pathology licensing laws (ASHA, 1981). And by the mid-1990s, there were so many paraprofessionals employed in speech-language pathology that ASHA developed a plan for credentialing them (ASHA, 1996).

The use of paraprofessionals in audiology does not appear to be as widespread as that in speech-language pathology. They certainly could be trained to do basic audiometric testing and hearing aid maintenance. Perhaps employment opportunities for audiology assistants will increase sufficiently in the future for ASHA to be motivated to credential them.

Several titles have been used for speech-language pathology paraprofessionals, including communication aide, speech-language pathology aide, and speech-language pathology assistant. Speech-language pathology assistant (SLPA) is the title that was being used by ASHA when this chapter was written.

SPEECH-LANGUAGE PATHOLOGISTS' CONCERNS ABOUT THE UTILIZATION OF SLPAs

Speech-language pathologists were expressing a number of concerns about the use of speech-language pathology assistants in articles and letters to the editor in ASHA publications and elsewhere when this chapter was written (e.g., Wolf, 1995). Among those mentioned most frequently were the following:

- It is demeaning to our profession to have paraprofessionals provide some services.
- Employers will hire paraprofessionals rather than speech-language pathologists because they can pay them a lower salary.
- A paraprofessional cannot provide the quality of service that a speech-language pathologist can provide.
- Speech-language pathology assistants will not be supervised adequately.
- Speech-language pathology assistants will exceed their scope of practice.
- The image of the profession will be degraded if the public believes that competent services can be provided by a person who has had only two years of training.

Each of these concerns will be dealt with in this section.

The first of these concerns is that it is demeaning to our profession to have paraprofessionals provide some services. This would be a valid concern if it wasn't standard practice in most other health-care professions to have paraprofessionals provide some of the routine services that do not require the training of a professional to perform competently. This, of course, is not the case. Nurse-practitioners and physician's assistants, for example, provide some such services for physicians. And physical therapy assistants and occupational therapy assistants do so for physical therapists and occupational therapists. The general public as well as other health-care professionals tend to expect routine tasks that do not require the expertise and training of a health-care professional to be done by a paraprofessional. They may, in fact, consider it demeaning for a professional to have to perform them.

Another concern is that employers will hire paraprofessionals rather than speech-language pathologists because they can pay them a lower

salary. It is possible that they will hire fewer speech-language pathologists than they would if SLPAs were not available. However, there probably will still be a large demand for speech-language pathologists, who
will be needed both to supervise SLPAs and to provide services that
SLPAs aren't competent to provide. While physical therapy assistants
and occupational therapy assistants have existed for a number of years,
there is still a large demand for physical therapists and occupational therapists! It can be argued, in fact, that the use of SLPAs can increase the employment opportunities for speech-language pathologists because they
are needed to supervise them and because a mix of speech-language
pathologists and SLPAs may make some clinical programs affordable
(fundable) that wouldn't be otherwise.

A third concern is that a paraprofessional cannot provide the quality
of service that a speech-language pathologist can provide. This concern
would certainly be valid if SLPAs were used to provide services that they
had not been trained to provide competently and/or if the services that
they provided were not adequately supervised. However, this would not
be a valid concern if SLPAs were only used to provide routine services
they had been trained to provide competently and the clinical services
they provided were adequately supervised. Years ago, there were few
dental hygienists and dentists cleaned teeth. While dental hygienists certainly have less training than dentists, they are able to do routine clean-
ing of teeth as well.

A fourth concern is that SLPAs will not be supervised adequately.
This concern is a real one. I have been told by several SLPAs that they received no real supervision. Without adequate supervision, the quality of
the service that SLPAs provide is likely to be lower than that provided by
speech-language pathologists. It is the ethical responsibility of speech-
language pathologists who have SLPAs to provide adequate supervision.

A fifth concern is that SLPAs will exceed their scope of practice. This
concern is also a real one. The SLPAs who told me that they weren't adequately supervised also told me that they were asked to do tasks that they
weren't trained to do competently. It is the ethical responsibility of
speech-language pathologists who have SLPAs to not only provide adequate supervision but to not require them to do tasks that they have not
been trained to do competently—ones that lie outside of their scope of
practice.

A sixth concern is that the image of the profession will be degraded if
the public believes that competent services can be provided by a person

who has had only two years of training. This does not appear to be a valid concern. The public has had enough experience with paraprofessionals to be aware that they are support personnel and are only competent to perform routine tasks under the supervision of a professional. To avoid their misleading the public, their title—"Speech-Language Pathology Assistant"—should appear on their name tag.

IS THERE REALLY A NEED FOR SLPAs?

The fact that paraprofessionals in speech-language pathology have been employed in educational and medical settings for more than twenty years indicates that they are meeting a real need. Incidentally, the fact that SLPAs have been available for more than twenty years and the job market for speech-language pathologists during most of this period has been excellent suggests that SLPAs are not the huge threat to the employment of speech-language pathologists that some speech-language pathologists consider them to be.

The employment of SLPAs can be helpful to both speech-language pathologists and those who pay for their services. The employment of SLPAs enables speech-language pathologists to devote more of their time to tasks that utilize their training and skills—tasks that tend to be challenging rather than being routine and run-of-the-mill. This increases the probability that they will maintain enthusiasm for their work—that is, it reduces the probability that they will burn out. The use of SLPAs may also enable them to offer services that would be too expensive to be fundable otherwise. And as I have indicated elsewhere, the use of SLPAs can enable some services to be provided more cost-effectively, which is an outcome that is regarded as highly desirable by administrators in both medical and public school settings.

HOW DOES THE SCOPE OF RESPONSIBILITIES FOR SLPAs DIFFER FROM THAT FOR SPEECH-LANGUAGE PATHOLOGISTS?

The scope of responsibilities for SLPAs differs considerably from that for speech-language pathologist. The American Speech-Language-Hearing

Association's Legislative Council in 1995 approved the following tasks for delegation to the SLPAs (ASHA, 1996):

- Conduct speech-language screenings (without interpretation) following specified screening protocols developed by the supervising speech-language pathologist.
- Provide direct treatment assistance to patients/clients identified by the supervising speech-language pathologist.
- Follow documented treatment plans or protocols developed by the supervising speech-language pathologist.
- Document patient/client progress toward meeting established objectives as stated in the treatment plan, and report this information to the supervising speech-language pathologist.
- Assist the speech-language pathologist during assessment of patients/clients, such as those who are difficult to test.
- Assist with informal documentation (e.g., tallying data for the speech-language pathologist to use), prepare materials, and assist with other clerical duties as directed by the speech-language pathologist.
- Schedule activities, prepare charts, records, graphs, or otherwise display data.
- Perform checks and maintenance of equipment.
- Participate with the speech-language pathologist in research projects, in-service training, and public relations programs.

The SLPA is not permitted to perform any of these tasks without the express knowledge and approval of the supervising speech-language pathologist.

The guidelines approved by the ASHA Legislative Council (ASHA, 1996) also specify the following tasks that an SLPA may NOT do (i.e., only a speech-language pathologist can do them):

- Perform standardized or nonstandardized diagnostic tests, formal or informal evaluations, or interpret test results.
- Participate in parent conferences, case conferences, or any interdisciplinary team without the presence of the supervising speech-language pathologist or other ASHA-certified speech-language pathologist designated by the supervising speech-language pathologist.
- Provide patient/client or family counseling.

- Write, develop, or modify a patient/client's individualized treatment plan in any way.
- Assist with patients/clients without following the individualized treatment plan prepared by the speech-language pathologist or without access to supervision.
- Sign any formal documents (e.g., treatment plans, reimbursement forms, or reports; the assistant should sign or initial informal treatment notes for review and co-signature by the supervising professional).
- Select patients/clients for service.
- Discharge a patient/client from services.
- Disclose clinical or confidential information either orally or in writing to anyone not designated by the supervising speech-language pathologist.
- Make referrals for additional services.
- Communicate with patient/client, family, or others regarding any aspect of the patient/client status or service without the specific consent of the supervising speech-language pathologist.
- Represent himself or herself as a speech-language pathologist.

Furthermore, these guidelines (ASHA, 1996) specify that the following are "exclusive responsibilities of the speech-language pathologist":

- Complete initial supervision training prior to accepting an assistant for supervision and upgrade supervision training on a regular basis.
- Participate in hiring the assistant.
- Document preservice training and credentials of the assistant.
- Inform patients/clients and families about the level (professional vs. support personnel), frequency, and duration of services as well as supervision.
- Represent the speech-language pathology team in all collaborative, interprofessional, interagency meetings, correspondence, and reports. This would not preclude the assistant from attending meetings along with the speech-language pathologist as a team member or drafting correspondence or reports for editing, approval, and signature by the speech-language pathologist.
- Make all clinical decisions including determining patient/client selection for inclusion in the caseload and dismissing patients/clients from treatment.

- Communicate with patients/clients, parents, and family members about diagnosis, prognosis, and treatment plan.
- Conduct diagnostic evaluations, assessments, or appraisals, and interpret obtained data in reports.
- Review each treatment plan with the assistant at least weekly.
- Delegate specific tasks to the assistant while retaining legal and ethical responsibility for all patient/client services provided or omitted.

One responsibility mentioned in this list—the first—creates a need for ongoing supervision training that will enable speech-language pathologists to utilize their SLPAs effectively for promoting the welfare of their clients/patients in ways that are unlikely to cause legal and/or ethical problems for either speech-language pathologists or SLPAs. There is definitely a need for such training. It was unclear when this chapter was written, however, exactly how such training will be provided. Until ASHA establishes relevant training programs, those speech-language pathologists who are required to supervise SLPAs may find books and workshops to be helpful that are intended to enable other health-care professionals to supervise paraprofessionals effectively, ethically, and with minimal risk of litigation.

NOTE: When this chapter was written, ASHA was in the process of formulating guidelines for supervising SLPAs. The tentative guidelines stated that speech-language pathologists should not supervise SLPAs until they have completed the ASHA certification examination, the Clinical Fellowship Year, and two additional years of clinical experience after receiving their Certificate of Clinical Competence in Speech-Language Pathology.

UTILIZING SLPAs EFFECTIVELY

Utilizing SLPAs effectively requires both an objective attitude toward using them and a degree of shrewdness.

An objective attitude toward utilizing SLPAs has several aspects. The first, and perhaps most important, is accepting the fact that the occupation of SLPA already exists. The question "Should there be speech-language pathology assistants?" is no longer a meaningful one to ask. It has already been answered. SLPAs are here and have been for more than twenty years. ASHA's motivation to credential SLPAs is more an attempt to remedy an existing situation (an absence of acceptable standards for training and supervising them) than it is to create a new one.

A second aspect of having an objective attitude toward utilizing SLPAs is accepting the fact that they are here to stay. The cost-containment philosophy that makes the use of SLPAs attractive to administrators in both medical and educational settings is unlikely to be discarded.

A third aspect of having an objective attitude toward SLPAs is regarding them as an asset rather than a liability—that is, regarding them as a vehicle for enhancing (rather than reducing) the quality of services your clients receive. If you regard them as an asset, you will tend to devote more energy to finding ways to use them effectively than to finding ways to avoid using them. Reports in the speech-language pathology literature indicate that they can be an asset (e.g., Harrison, 1995; Jimenez & Iseyama, 1987; Werven, 1992).

In addition to needing an objective attitude to use SLPAs appropriately, you will also need to be shrewd. You will have to develop a mindset that will enable you to spot tasks your SLPA(s) can do competently that can directly promote the welfare of the persons whom you serve professionally and also do so indirectly by relieving you of responsibilities that don't require your level of training, thereby giving you more time for tasks that do require it. You will also have to develop an awareness of the amount of supervision that a particular SLPA will require to do particular tasks competently. Your goal will be to provide the appropriate amount of supervision. If you provide too little, tasks may not be performed competently. And if you provide too much (i.e., you attempt to micro-manage their activities), it will both take time away from your other responsibilities and interfere with your developing a good working relationship. None of us give our best efforts to people who appear to regard us as being stupid! If a task would require considerable supervision long-term for it to be done by an SLPA, it may be neither sensible nor cost-effective to assign the task to an SLPA.

LEGAL IMPLICATIONS OF THE RELATIONSHIP BETWEEN THE SLPA AND THE SPEECH-LANGUAGE PATHOLOGIST

The relationship between the speech-language pathologist and the SLPA is legally designated metaphorically as a "master-servant" one. In this type of relationship, the "master's" responsibilities include both assigning tasks to the "servant" and telling him or her how to perform them. If the "master" assigns inappropriate tasks to the "servant" and/or inadequately instructs the "servant" in how to perform them and as a result someone is harmed, the "master" is held at least partially responsible. In paraprofessional-professional relationships, such harm may be viewed by a court as resulting from negligence, thereby constituting *malpractice* (see Chapter 5). Consequently, it is necessary for speech-language pathologists to select appropriate tasks for SLPAs and supervise their doing them adequately not only to meet the ethical requirements for ASHA certification and state licensure, but also to avoid becoming involved in malpractice litigation.

REFERENCES

American Speech-Language-Hearing Association (1970). Guidelines on the role, training, and supervision of the communication aide. *Asha*, 12(2), 78–80.

American Speech-Language-Hearing Association. (1981). Employment and utilization of supportive personnel in audiology and speech-language pathology. *Asha*, 23(3), 165–169.

American Speech-Language-Hearing Association (1996). Guidelines for the training, credentialing, use, and supervision of speech-language pathology assistants. *Asha*, 38 (Supplement 16), 21–34.

Harrison, F. H. (November/December, 1995). Debate continues. *Asha*, 37.

Jimenez, B., & Iseyama, D. (1987). A model for training and using communication assistants. *Language, Speech, and Hearing Services in Schools*, 18 (2), 168–171.

Werven, G. (August, 1992). Training support personnel to provide services to persons with head injury. *Asha*, 34, 72–74.

Wolf, K. E. (November/December, 1995). Speech-language pathology assistants: Support personnel or lower-level practitioners? *Asha*, 37, 45.

▶ 11

Documenting Treatment Efficacy

All speech-language pathologists and audiologists should be motivated to document the efficacy of treatment on their clients. There are a number of reasons why they should want to do this type of documentation. These are discussed in this chapter and some guidelines are presented. The chapter ends with a plea for clinicians to contribute to the profession's outcome database and a description of some ways by which you may be able to do so.

WHAT IS TREATMENT EFFICACY DOCUMENTATION?

Documenting treatment efficacy can be defined as "an ongoing, unbroken stream of activity seeking to prove the effectiveness of clinical procedures" (ASHA, 1995, p. 37). To document the efficacy of a particular treatment, it is necessary to answer the following four questions with data that possess adequate levels of validity, reliability, and generality (ASHA, 1995, p. 38):

- What was achieved?
- How long did it take?
- How much did it cost?
- Did it make a difference?

Being able to answer these questions will enhance your ability to compete successfully for shrinking health-care and K–12 education dollars.

To document treatment efficacy until fairly recently it was usually only necessary to answer the first of these questions: "What was achieved?" Merely documenting that a treatment produced a measurable change was often adequate to establish its efficacy. This is no longer true. Once it has been established that a treatment produces a measurable change (or changes), it is then necessary to document that the observed change (or changes) can enable a client to function sufficiently better in the "real world" to justify the cost of the treatment. A treatment for which there is solid documentation that it can enable a client to function significantly better in the "real world" is more likely to be funded than for one for which there is no such documentation. And a treatment that is likely to result in a "real-world" benefit to a client is more likely to be funded if its cost is relatively low than if it is relatively high. What we have here is the utilization of the same cost/benefit ratio that is commonly used for making business decisions. It is being used here because the persons who write the guidelines for making treatment funding decisions are mostly MBA-types.

For your answers to these four questions to be likely to be viewed by others as trustworthy, the data that were used to answer the questions would have to be regarded by them as possessing adequate levels of validity, reliability, and generality. The *validity* of the data used to answer a question refers to their *appropriateness* for doing so. To determine, for example, how many sessions/hours tend to be needed to complete a particular treatment in a medical setting, using billing data would probably be appropriate for doing so.

The *reliability* of the data used to answer a question refers to its *repeatability*. To determine, for example, whether the billing data used to specify how many sessions/hours tend to be needed to complete a particular treatment in a medical setting is reliable, a second person could be asked to abstract the same data (or a sample of it) from the files. The two sets would then be compared. If the second set corresponded very closely to the first, then the observations would be repeatable and consequently, they would be reliable.

The *generality* of the data used to answer a question refers to the extent to which the events observed are *representative* of those designated by the question. Inferences about the efficacy of a treatment based on observations of a client in the therapy room may be inaccurate because the client behaves differently there than he or she does in the "real world." Assuming that the question the data was being used to answer pertained to the "real world," the level of generality of such inferences would be uncertain.

For further information about validity, reliability and generality as they relate to sets of data used for answering questions, see Chapter 12 of Silverman (1998).

POSSIBLE BENEFITS FROM DOCUMENTING TREATMENT EFFICACY

What benefits can a clinician derive from documenting treatment efficacy? One such benefit would be enabling him or her to function in a manner that is consistent with the Code of Ethics of the American Speech-Language-Hearing Association. The current (1998) version of the Code states that "individuals shall evaluate services rendered to determine effectiveness." Consequently, for clinicians to function ethically they must systematically evaluate the impacts of the services they render.

There are a number of benefits in addition to satisfying the requirements of the ASHA Ethical Code that you can derive from documenting treatment efficacy. The following are several of them.

- It will tend to make your job more stimulating and less routine. What you learn is likely to motivate you to try to increase your treatment efficacy, thereby reducing the probability that you will burn out from boredom.
- It will help to satisfy your employer's demand for *accountability*. Almost all speech-language pathologists and audiologists are required by their employers to document the efficacy of their treatments for funding and other purposes.
- It should help you to become a more effective clinician by motivating you to discard or modify treatments that do not tend to be helpful to your clients.
- It will enable you to contribute to the body of information on treatment efficacy that speech-language pathologists and audiologists must have to compete successfully for health-care and K–12 education-related dollars. The need for this type of database and how clinicians can contribute to it is dealt with in depth elsewhere in the chapter.

This list of possible benefits from documenting treatment efficacy is not exhaustive. There undoubtedly are other ways in which a clinician could benefit from doing it.

TREATMENT EFFICACY DOCUMENTATION AS CLINICAL RESEARCH

Most clinicians don't think of themselves as doing clinical research when they are documenting the impacts of treatments on clients. Rather, they think of themselves as determining if their clients are closer to achieving specific goals than they were at earlier points in time and if they are closer to achieving them, by how much. What they are actually doing for each such goal is attempting to answer one or both of the following questions:

1. Is the client any closer to achieving the goal than he or she was on an earlier date (perhaps the date that treatment began)?
2. If the answer to the first question is yes, how much closer is the client to achieving the goal?

They, of course, will want to use a methodology for answering these questions that will maximize the likelihood that their answers would be accurate. The methodology that is most likely to enable them to achieve their objective (i.e., accurate answers) is referred to as the *scientific method*.

The scientific method can be viewed as set of rules for asking and answering questions. Using these rules to answer questions, as I have indicated previously, maximizes the odds that the answers will be correct. This is the reason why investigators in all fields use methodologies for answering research questions that follow the rules of the scientific method.

Documenting treatment efficacy can be viewed as doing clinical research. Doing clinical research involves answering clinically relevant questions using methodologies that (at least hopefully) do not violate any of the rules of the scientific method.

Why might it be beneficial for clinicians to view documenting treatment efficacy as doing clinical research? There are several ways that they and the persons whom they serve professionally could benefit from their doing so. First, it could provide them with an additional source of methodological information. While the literature on methodology for "documenting treatment efficacy" is relatively small, that which deals with answering clinical research questions using a *single-subject design* is relatively large (see Silverman, 1998). Consequently, viewing it in this way can enable a clinician to benefit from the methodological research and advice in both the treatment efficacy documentation literature and the single-subject clinical research literature. This, incidentally, highlights the need for clinicians to be trained to be producers as well as consumers of clinical research. The assumption that it is unnecessary for clinicians to know how to do clinical research because very few of them are expected by their employer to do it is no longer valid. Doing a type of clinical research—documenting treatment outcome—is a responsibility mentioned in the job description of most (if not all) speech-language pathologists and audiologists.

Another way that the persons whom speech-language pathologists and audiologists serve professionally could benefit from their viewing documenting treatment efficacy as doing clinical research is by motivating them to contribute to the body of knowledge on treatment efficacy. One of the rules of the scientific method states that questions, answers, and interpretations should be communicated to anyone who could benefit from knowing them. Consequently, questions, answers, and interpretations that are viewed as clinical research tend to be reported at professional meetings, in professional journals and newsletters, and on clinically related sites on the Internet. At least some of the data that clinicians in our field gather as a part of their responsibility for treatment efficacy documentation could be helpful to others. Therefore, their viewing this responsibility as a clinical research one could motivate them to share their data with others and doing so could also provide a justification for sharing it with others that their employer would accept.

CONSIDERATIONS FOR DOCUMENTING TREATMENT EFFICACY

Since documenting treatment efficacy is doing clinical research, the research design considerations for doing it are those scientific-method-related ones to which attention must be paid when answering research questions to maximize the odds of a correct answer. Specifically, they are the ones to which attention must be paid when doing single-subject research. There are a number of articles and books that deal with single-subject research design considerations, including Silverman (1998).

CONTRIBUTING TO THE PROFESSION'S DATABASE FOR EFFICACY DOCUMENTATION

Our survival as a profession will depend in large part on our ability to secure funding for our services from third-party payers. Such third-party payers include departments of public instruction and medical insurance programs. Since their ability to fund clinical services is limited (and is likely to continue being so in the future), they will be investing most of their resources in treatments for which there is documentation for their efficacy. In particular, they will be investing in treatments for which there is documentation that they are likely to enable people to function better in the "real world." That is, they will be investing in treatments that enable those who receive them to cope more successfully with whatever they have to cope with in their environment. Consequently, the stronger the evidence for the efficacy of a treatment, the more likely the treatment is to be approved for funding by medical insurance programs and/or departments of public instruction.

For the reasons that I have indicated, it is in the self-interest of all speech-language pathologists and audiologists to augment (strengthen) the available documentation for the efficacy of their treatments. That is, it is in their self-interest to contribute to the treatment efficacy database for our field. They can do this by making the efficacy data that they gather on their clients for their employer available to others in the field. They, of course, would have to do this in a way that maintains client confidentiality. And for the data they share to be likely to strengthen the documentation for the efficacy of certain treatments, the data would have to be gathered in a manner that is consistent with the rules of the scientific method. That is, the data would have to be gathered in a manner that is likely to yield adequate levels of validity, reliability, and generality for answering the efficacy questions that they will be used to answer.

The treatment efficacy database for our field is a virtual rather than an actual one. It consists of sets of data that can contribute to answering one or more of the four efficacy questions for particular treatments (listed elsewhere in the chapter). The sets of data that can help to answer a particular question for a particular treatment may be combined by an inferential statistical procedure known as meta-analysis (see Chapter 10 in Silverman, 1998). Meta-analysis has been widely used to merge sets of data for documenting psychotherapy and other types of treatment efficacy. The fact that meta-analysis is a statistical procedure that is consistent with the rules of the scientific method would tend to enhance the credibility of the answers it yields to third-party payers and others.

Clinicians can contribute the documentation data they gather to the treatment efficacy database in several ways. They can do so by presenting them at professional meetings, by "posting" them on Internet bulletin boards, and by reporting them in professional newsletters and journals. The latter is usually the best way because it is likely to make data available to more clinicians than are the others.

REFERENCES

American Speech-Language-Hearing Association. (November/December, 1995). Collecting outcome data. *Asha, 37,* 36–38.

Silverman, F. H. (1998). *Research Design and Evaluation in Speech-Language Pathology and Audiology* (4th ed.). Boston: Allyn & Bacon.

▶ 12

Patient (Client) Rights

Patients (clients) have certain rights that are recognized by both the courts and ethical practices boards. If you fail to make them aware of or deny them any of these rights, you can be sued and/or lose your license or certification. Consequently, it is crucial that you know what these rights are and how to cope with them appropriately. We will focus in this chapter on certain of these right that are relevant for the practice of speech-language pathology and audiology. Since most statements of these rights refer to persons served professionally as patients rather than clients, we will do so also in this chapter. Be aware, however, that the persons whom we serve professionally have these right regardless of whether we refer to them as patients or clients.

SOURCES OF PATIENT RIGHTS

The two primary promulgators of patient rights are legislatures and courts. Successful suits alleging violations of patient rights can strengthen previously accepted rights or establish new ones. And unsuccessful suits of this type can raise questions about the enforceability of previously accepted rights. Consequently, the rights that the courts recognize a patient has at one point in time may not be identical to those that they recognize a patient has at another. For this reason, it isn't possible to present a complete list of patient rights.

While the rights patients have that are recognized by the courts change from time to time, there are some that the courts have recognized for many years and are likely to continue doing so. These are the rights on which we will focus in this chapter.

A PATIENT'S "BILL OF RIGHTS"

Health-care professionals have an obligation to inform patients about their rights. Some health-care professionals refer to the document that they use to do so as a patient's "bill of rights." To assist health-care workers in formulating such bills of rights, the Joint Commission on Accreditation of Healthcare Organizations (JCAHO) issued a compilation of patient rights. According to Breske (1994, p. 14), these rights can be summarized as follows:

- The right to a reasonable response to requests/needs for treatment or service
- The right to considerate and respectful care
- The right to make decisions, in collaboration with the physician [and other involved health-care workers], involving health care
- The right to information necessary to make treatment decisions that reflect wishes
- The right to information at admission on grievance procedures and specific patient rights
- The right to participate in discussion of ethical issues
- The right to be informed of any human experimentation or research affecting treatment
- The right to personal privacy within law's limits and to personal privacy and confidentiality of information
- The right of the patient's guardian, next of kin, or authorized person to delineate the patient's wishes should he or she become incapable.

In the remainder of this chapter we explore some of the implications that each of these rights has for speech-language pathologists and audiologists.

The Right to a Reasonable Response to Requests/Needs for Treatment or Service

This right has a number of implications for speech-language pathologists and audiologists, including the following:

- Patients must be scheduled for evaluation within a reasonable period of time or given the option of being referred elsewhere.
- Following evaluation, patients must be scheduled for treatment within a reasonable period of time or given the option of being referred elsewhere.
- Requests for copies of reports to be sent to other professionals must be complied with within a reasonable period of time.
- Requests for second opinions and other referrals must be complied with within a reasonable period of time.
- The reason(s) for not honoring a patient's request for treatments or services must be given and if the patient challenges the decision, he or she must be informed about procedures for appealing it.
- A patient of another health-care professional (e.g., a physician) who requests a referral to a speech-language pathologist or audiologist has a right to receive a prompt response to his or her request.
- A patient who requests funding for speech-language pathology or audiology services from a third-party payer has a right to receive a prompt response to his or her request.

The Right to Considerate and Respectful Care

This right has significant implications that may not be obvious, including the following:

- The clinician must be sensitive to and respect any attitude toward treatment a patient has that arises from his or her cultural background and differs from the clinician's attitude toward it (see Chapter 14).
- The clinician should be on time for appointments.
- The clinician should really "listen" to what the patient has to say.
- The clinician should not communicate with the patient in a manner that is condescending or patronizing.

- The clinician should involve the patient and possibly his or her family in the treatment planning process if the patient is not a young child or an adult who is severely cognitively impaired.
- The clinician should answer any treatment and prognosis-related questions honestly.

The Right to Make Decisions, in Collaboration with the Physician [and Other Involved Health-Care Workers], Involving Health Care

The patient has the final word with regard to his or her health care or that of his or her minor children (assuming that the patient has legal custody of them). He or she has the right to refuse to accept any or all of your recommendations for treatment. And he or she has the right to pursue treatment options that you don't recommend. You, of course, are not obliged to provide treatments that you don't recommend. It may, in fact, be a violation of the ASHA Ethical Code for you to do so.

The Right to Information Necessary to Make Treatment Decisions That Reflect Wishes

Your patients need information to make informed treatment decisions. They have a right to expect you to provide sufficient information about treatment options to enable them to make such decisions. You should describe the various treatment options as objectively as you can. You, of course, should indicate which one (or ones) you recommend and your reasons for doing so.

There is another reason why it is crucial to fully inform your patients about treatment options, including any risks associated with them. Failure to do so can negate a patient's *informed consent* for treatment and consequently, it can make you vulnerable to litigation by the patient and/or his or her family. A patient's or legal guardian's signature on a consent form will not provide legal protection if there is no documentation for the patient or guardian having been fully informed about potential risks before signing it. Consequently, a description of such risks should appear on the consent form.

The Right to Information at Admission on Grievance Procedures and Specific Patient Rights

The patient should be informed of his or her rights before beginning treatment as well as whom to contact if he or she believes that any them have been ignored. Your school or medical facility will hopefully employ someone whose responsibilities include attempting to resolve grievances. Patients can be informed of their rights and grievance procedures in several ways, one of which is to hand them a brochure containing the information as a part of your admission procedure. Another is to print it as a poster and mount it on the wall of your waiting room and/or the wall of some other room where patients are likely to see it.

The Right to Participate in Discussion of Ethical Issues

If there is concern about whether treatment or its continuation is warranted for ethical reasons, the patient (or his or her family) has a right to participate in the discussion. The relevance of this right for speech-language pathologists and audiologists pertains mainly to conflicts between what a patient (or his or her family) desires and what the clinician believes he or she can provide without violating the ASHA Code of Ethics. A clinician, for example, may recommend discontinuing treatment because he or she considers it unlikely that a patient will benefit from further therapy. The patient or a member of his or her family who disagrees with the recommendation has the right to an opportunity to explain why he or she believes it is not in the patient's best interest to discontinue treatment and to attempt to have the recommendation withdrawn.

The Right to Be Informed of Any Human Experimentation or Research Affecting Treatment

There has been considerable interest since the Nuremburg trials, which were conducted after World War II for "crimes against humanity" committed by persons in Germany associated with the Third Reich (see Hoedeman, 1991), in the mental and physical welfare of persons who serve as subjects in research studies. This interest has resulted in the creation of regulations on both national and international levels that are intended to protect the rights of such persons. Consequently, if the treatment that a patient will be receiving could be regarded as "experimental" or if some of the data that the clinician collects from the patient while he or she is in treatment will be used for research purposes, the patient has a right to know and these regulations must be complied with—particularly the requirement to obtain the patient's (or his or her legal guardian's) informed consent. This requirement is spelled out in the World Health Association's *Declaration of Helsinki*:

> *If at all possible, consistent with patient psychology, the doctor [clinician] should obtain the patient's freely given consent after the patient has been given a full explanation. In case of legal incapacity, consent should also be procured from the legal guardian; in the case of physical incapacity, the permission of the legal guardian replaces that of the patient.* (Silverman, 1992, p. 217)

Securing a patient's *informed consent* for an "experimental" treatment can provide both you and your employer with some protection against litigation arising from allegations that the patient was physically or mentally harmed by it. If the patient was aware of a particular risk before consenting to receive the treatment and if he or she was harmed in a manner predictable from this risk, the patient would be unlikely to be successful if he or she sued either you or your employer.

One of the main types of litigation against which a patient's informed consent to receive an experimental treatment can provide some protection is *battery*. According to Fried:

> *The central concept of battery is the offense to personal dignity that occurs when another impinges on one's bodily integrity without full and valid consent. A punch in the stomach or being doused with a pail of water are classic examples. It is not necessary to show that one has been physically injured, much less that one has suffered financial loss. The injury is to dignity. That being the case, law suits have been brought and won against doctors who performed needed and successful operations, but without consent of their patients.* (1974, p. 15)

Consequently, subjecting patients to treatment programs (particularly experimental ones) without their "full and valid consent" can result in litigation for battery even if they were not injured.

The requirement that must be satisfied to justify intentionally invading another's bodily integrity is securing his or her *free and informed* consent to do so. According to Fried:

> *To be effective the consent must be to the particular contact with the person in question, and if procured by "fraud or mistake as to the essential character" of the conduct it is invalid. . . . And it is not just active fraud or concealment which destroys consent. The doctor [clinician] who obtains consent has the duty to give the facts the patient needs to make an informed choice. . . . He must tell the patient about the benefits and risks of the treatment and how likely they are. And some courts have said that the patient must also be told about the hazards and advantages of alternative forms of treatment.* (1974, pp. 19–20)

Consequently, for a patient's consent for treatment to be regarded by a court as having been *free and informed,* the clinician would have to be able to prove that the patient was not coerced into giving it and that the patient had been fully informed (i.e., had not been deceived) about the risks involved before he or she gave it.

Under some circumstances a patient's free and informed consent to receive an experimental treatment may not be essential. One such circumstance would be when the subject is a *child*, particularly a very young child who would be unable to understand the treatment and consequently, would be incapable of giving informed consent. Consent in such a circumstance would have to be obtained from the child's legal guardian, who in most instances would be a parent. However, a guardian's ability to consent to a child's receiving such a treatment is limited:

> *The tendency of the law has been to limit what may be done to children and incompetents just because they are unable to give effective consent. And those who act for them are strictly charged to act only in the manifest interests of these persons.* (Fried, 1974, p. 23)

The message here is that securing a guardian's consent for his or her child to receive an experimental treatment would not always provide protection against litigation, particularly if a legitimate question could be raised about it having been in the child's best interest to have received the treatment.

A patient's free and informed consent also may not be essential if he or she is an adult whom the court would classify as *incompetent*. Adults are likely to be classified as incompetent if they are thought to be unable to make rational decisions regarding their own welfare. Persons diagnosed as psychotic or severely mentally retarded are likely to be classified as incompetent. Persons who are severely communicatively handicapped (e.g., global aphasics) may also be classified as incompetent. A court-appointed guardian could consent to such a person receiving a particular treatment. The restrictions on such a guardian's ability to do so are the same as for guardians of children.

The Right to Personal Privacy within Law's Limits and to Personal Privacy and Confidentiality of Information

A patient has a right to expect any information that he or she gives a clinician orally or in writing to be treated as confidential under *almost all circumstances*. A patient also has a right to expect any reports that are written about him or her to be treated as confidential *under most circumstances*. The words "under most circumstances" were italicized because this right is not absolute. There are several circumstances—such as information or documents being subpoenaed by a court—when a clinician is required to divulge personal information.

To what specific circumstances does the right to personal privacy and confidentiality of information apply? There are a number, including the following:

- The communication of information to other professionals in reports. The patient's (or legal guardian's) written consent is almost always required to do so.
- Patient records in filing cabinets and in computer databases must be safeguarded from unauthorized and unnecessary access. Only persons who have a legitimate reason to access such information should be able to do so and the information they are able to access should be only what they require. Persons who need information from patient records for billing purposes, for example, should only be able to access the specific information they need. If patient records are kept in a computer database, the database should be multiple-level password protected; if a database has this feature, the ability of billing department personnel to view patient records can be limited by giving them a password that restricts their access to information they need for billing purposes.

- Recordings (audio or video) of treatment sessions cannot be made and used for any purpose without the written consent of the patient or his or her legal guardian. Furthermore, no one (e.g., students) can be allowed to observe their treatment (either in the therapy room or through a one-way mirror) without written permission.
- Patients' photographs and/or names cannot be used for marketing purposes without their or their legal guardians' written permission.
- Articles that contain information about a patient's treatment cannot be published without the patient's (or his or her legal guardian's) written permission if there is any possibility that the patient could be recognized from the information provided.

The Right of the Patient's Guardian, Next of Kin, or Authorized Person to Delineate the Patient's Wishes Should He or She Become Incapable

If a patient has communicated certain wishes regarding treatment to family or other authorized persons before losing the ability to communicate, the patient has a right to have his or her wishes honored. They may be communicated by a *living will* and, of course, can include wishes that pertain to the treatment of a patient's swallowing or communicative disorder. Such wishes are likely to place restrictions on treatment.

REFERENCES

Breske, S. (February, 1994). JCAHO established 'bill of rights' for patients. *Advance/Rehabilitation*, 14, 16–17.

Fried, C. (1974). *Medical Experimentation: Personal Integrity and Social Policy*. New York: American Elsevier.

Hoedeman, P. (1991). *Hitler or Hippocrates: Medical Experiments and Euthanasia in the Third Reich*. Sussex, England: The Book Guild.

Silverman, F. H. (1992). *Legal/Ethical Considerations, Restrictions, and Obligations for Clinicians Who Treat Communicative Disorders*. Springfield, IL: Charles C. Thomas.

▶ 13

Scope of Practice Issues and Keeping up to Date

The scope of practice for speech-language pathologists and audiologists has changed from time to time during this century and is likely to continue doing so. It has, in fact, changed dramatically during the forty years I've been a speech-language pathologist. When I began my career, for example, the scope of practice of speech-language pathologists did not include augmentative communication. It wasn't officially recognized by ASHA as being within their scope of practice until the late 1970s. The same is true for swallowing—dysphagia—therapy. While patients who have dysphagia now make up a significant percentage of the caseloads of many (perhaps most) speech-language pathologists who are employed in hospitals and nursing homes, few (if any) speech-language pathologists treated patients for dysphagia when I entered the field. In the public schools when I entered the field, the majority of the children treated by speech-language pathologists had an articulation disorder—now most of them have a language disorder. These are just a few of the ways that the scope of practice of speech-language pathologists has changed during the forty years I've been in the field.

The scope of practice of audiologists has also changed dramatically during the past forty years. For example, at the beginning of this period very few audiologists dispensed hearing aids. Now most of them do so.

Regardless of whether you are a speech-language pathologist or audiologist, the scope of practice for your field is likely to change (at least a little) during your professional career. This "certainty" has a number of implications, several of which will be explored in this chapter.

HOW SCOPE OF PRACTICE CHANGES

ASHA periodically redefines the scope of practice for both speech-language pathologists and audiologists. Does a change in the definition *cause* a change in their practice or *recognize* a change that has already occurred? This is a "Which came first, the chicken or the egg?" kind of question. In at least a few instances, a change in the ASHA scope-of-practice definition undoubtedly recognized a change that had already occurred. Below are three examples of a change in ASHA's definition recognizing an existing change in practice.

Myofunctional Therapy

In the early 1960s, many speech-language pathologists began treating cases of tongue-thrust (reverse swallowing) for orthodontists. This, incidentally, was one of the first times when speech-language pathologists were viewed as competent by practitioners outside the field to treat disorders of the mouth that do not necessarily adversely affect speech. ASHA did not redefine the scope of practice of speech-language pathologists to include myofunctional therapy until many years later.

Augmentative Communication

Speech-language pathologists began using augmentative communication strategies and aids with severely communicatively impaired children and adults during the 1960s. However, it wasn't until the late 1970s that ASHA formed an ad hoc committee to begin to define the scope of practice for speech-language pathologists with regard to these strategies and aids.

Supervision of Speech-Language Pathology Assistants

Paraprofessionals in speech-language pathology have been functioning in public school and medical settings under the supervision of speech-language pathologists since the 1970s (and possibly before). However, it wasn't until the 1990s that ASHA added supervising speech-language pathology assistants to its statement that defines scope of practice for speech-language pathologists.

WHY SCOPE OF PRACTICE CHANGES

What factors cause the scope of practice for speech-language pathologists and audiologists to change? There are a number of factors that singly or in combination can produce such changes. Some of them are described in this section. The order in which factors are discussed is not intended to suggest their importance.

Multiskilling

The multiskilling initiative has resulted in speech-language pathologists and audiologists assuming responsibilities that are not specified in ASHA's scope of practice definitions for their fields (Pietranton & Lynch, 1995). With multiskilling, persons are "cross-trained to provide more than one function, often in more than one discipline" (Pietranton & Lynch, 1995, p. 38). Some of the tasks that have been assigned to speech-language pathologists and audiologists are ordinarily performed by persons in other disciplines. An example of such a task that was being done by some local speech-language pathologists when this chapter was written is deep suctioning the respiratory tracts of their patients. Such suctioning, when needed, ordinarily is done by a respiratory therapist. It seems likely that at least some of the responsibilities that speech-language pathologists and audiologists have assumed through multiskilling will eventually be added to their scopes of practice by ASHA.

New Devices

The development of new devices for assessment and treatment has expanded the scopes of practice of both speech-language pathologists and audiologists. The development of augmentative communication aids, for example, resulted in speech-language pathologists treating persons whom they probably would not have treated otherwise—that is, severely speech-impaired people who have a poor prognosis for improving speech.

Changes in the ASHA Code of Ethics

During the 1970s and earlier, it was a violation of the ASHA ethical code for audiologists to dispense hearing aids for profit. When ASHA modified this aspect of the Code, the scope of practice for audiologists expanded dramatically.

Federal Legislation

Congress has passed bills (and is likely to continue doing so) that mandate services for persons previously unserved or underserved. Some provisions of these bills have added to the scopes of practice of both speech-language pathologists and audiologists. Examples of populations that have been added to the scope of practice of speech-language pathologists by Congress in recent years include the "zero to three" and neonatal populations.

Unfilled Niches

Both speech-language pathologists and audiologists have expanded their scopes of practice by treating functional disorders of the mouth and ears that were not being treated by other health-care professionals. Doing so, of course, required them to get additional training. A relatively recent example of speech-language pathologists expanding their scope of practice by niche filling is their increasing involvement with dysphagia (swallowing) therapy.

COPING WITH A CHANGING SCOPE OF PRACTICE

The need for speech-language pathologists and audiologists to accept the challenge of coping with a changing scope of practice is not new. Practitioners in both fields have had to do it frequently to survive during the past fifty years. The changes that have occurred in their scopes of practice during the past ten years have been at least as great as those that occurred during the previous forty years. Consequently, it is highly likely that you will have to cope with such changes throughout your professional career.

There are a number of factors that could influence your ability to successfully cope with such changes. Three of the more important ones that are likely to be under your control (at least partially) are discussed in this section.

Your Ability to Recognize the Need for Change and to View It as a Challenge Rather Than a Tragedy

Contemplating change tends to precipitate anxiety. This is true even for changes that are highly likely to enrich your life. To experience anxiety while contemplating change is to be human! It is not abnormal!

Some persons cope with such anxiety by either refusing to recognize (i.e., denying) a need for change or by recognizing that a need to change exists but demanding a return to the status quo. A hospital-based speech-language pathologist would be refusing to recognize such a need by failing to conform to the requirement of the managed health-care philosophy (see Chapter 9) to treat patients in the way that can both meet their needs and be cost-effective. A speech-language pathologist, for example, may resist using a speech-language pathology assistant (see Chapter 10) for doing routine tasks when doing so would enable the speech-language pathologist to provide certain services more cost-effectively without sacrificing quality.

Another way that a person may attempt to cope with change-related anxiety is by recognizing that a change has occurred (or is occurring) but demanding that it be nullified—that there be a return to "the good old days." Letters to the editor, for example, have appeared in the *ASHA Leader* demanding that ASHA do something to neutralize aspects of the managed health-care philosophy that require speech-language pathologists and audiologists to change their modes of service delivery. Letters to the editor have also appeared in the *ASHA Leader* demanding that ASHA discourage the training and employment of speech-language pathology assistants.

There is no question that your survival as a clinician will depend, in large part, on your ability to anticipate, recognize, and cope with change. You must accept the fact that the ways in which you will be expected to provide services and the services that you will be expected to provide are far more likely to change from time to time during your professional career than to remain constant. In fact, the likelihood that they will remain constant throughout your professional career is probably close to that for winning your state's lottery. While your ability to keep change from occurring is limited at best, your ability to control how you react to the need for change is not. The ways in which you react to the need for change can affect your ability to cope successfully with it. If you deny the need for change or delay attempting to cope with change in the belief that the need to have to cope with it will be eliminated (i.e., there will be a return to the "good old days"), you will be placing your ability to survive professionally at risk. On the other hand, if you view the necessity to change positively—as offering you a challenge—not only will you be enhancing your ability to survive professionally, but you may also be reducing the likelihood of your burning out. One factor that undoubtedly can contribute to burnout is boredom. Successfully coping with "new realities" (i.e., meeting job-related challenges) is likely to make your job more stimulating intellectually.

Your Attitude toward Continuing Education

It is likely that you will have to acquire additional information and skills throughout your professional career if you are to cope successfully with a changing scope of practice. Like scope of practice not remaining constant, you can view your having to spend time on continuing education either positively or negatively—that is, as either offering an opportunity to engage in an activity that can benefit both you and your patients or as something you are required to do to maintain your license or certification that you probably would not do otherwise. These two attitudes define the ends of a continuum. Where along this continuum your attitude toward continuing education falls is likely to significantly influence your ability to cope successfully with a changing scope of practice.

Your attitude toward continuing education is likely to influence the amount of information you acquire. If you regard participating in continuing education as a chore (i.e., an activity you would avoid if you could), then you are likely to invest little of yourself in it. You are likely to merely "go through the motions"—do the minimum amount you have to do to get credit for participating. You are also likely to be resentful about having to spend time doing it. If, on the other hand, you assume that the information provided is necessary to cope successfully with a changing scope of practice, then you are likely to acquire it, thereby enhancing your ability to survive as a clinician.

Your attitude toward continuing education also influences the extent to which you are likely to modify your clinical functioning to meet the demands of a changing scope of practice. If you have a negative attitude toward continuing education, you are unlikely to invest as much of yourself in it, which would tend to result in your acquiring less information from it. Having less information would obviously impede your ability to meet these demands.

Your Ability to Acquire and Evaluate Information

Your ability to cope successfully with changes in your scope of practice, as I have indicated previously, will be partially determined by your ability to acquire needed information. What you may have to do to acquire such information can range from getting the answer to a question from a colleague to participating in a training program.

Your ability to cope successfully with changes in your scope of practice will also depend on your motivation and ability to evaluate the information you acquire for accuracy. Before using any such information, you will hopefully make a judgment about the amount of confidence you can have in its accuracy—that is, a judgment about whether its validity, reliability, and generality are likely to be adequate for your purpose. See Chapter 12 in Silverman (1998) for guidelines for performing such an evaluation.

OPTIONS FOR CONTINUING EDUCATION

Assuming that you want to invest in continuing education throughout your professional career, what options are available to you for doing so? I will attempt in this section to *partially* answer this question. I have emphasized the word "partially" for two reasons. First, there may currently be options for doing so other than those that I mention. And second, new options for doing so may become available in the future. One such option, the Internet, for example, only became a viable continuing education one for many clinicians during the 1990s.

The continuing education options currently available to speech-language pathologists and audiologists include the following:

- Workshops, seminars, inservice presentations, lectures, and short courses. These are offered under the auspices of colleges and universities, clinical facilities, vendors, and professional organizations such as ASHA and state speech-language-hearing associations. They range in duration from a few hours to a few weeks. Participants may be at a single site or at multiple sites that are linked by satellite and utilize "distance learning" technology. Participants may receive continuing education credit toward license/certification renewal and/or the ASHA ACE certificate.

- College/university courses. These would be courses offered for graduate credit. They may be conducted in a classroom, offered by correspondence, and/or presented utilizing some form of computer "distance learning" technology. They may be a requirement for a training program that culminates in the awarding of a degree or certificate (e.g., an AuD).
- Informal communication with peers. This is perhaps the main way that many speech-language pathologists and audiologists try to keep up to date. They share information with each other during informal conversations. They also do so by "snail" mail, e-mail, and by asking and answering questions on computer bulletin boards, such as the one that ASHA maintains on its web site.
- Attending professional association conventions. ASHA and most (if not all) state speech-language-hearing associations have an annual conventions. Almost all other professional associations to which speech-language pathologists or audiologists belong also have annual conventions. Their main function is to provide those attending with formal and informal opportunities for continuing education. The formal avenues include paper presentations, poster presentations, videotape presentations, short courses, miniseminars, scientific exhibits, and commercial exhibits. Informal avenues include opportunities to exchange information with peers during scheduled "social" events such as sight-seeing tours, cocktail hours, luncheons, and banquets. Some persons believe that they learn at least as much at conventions by exchanging information with peers as they do by attending sessions.
- Reading professional books, journals, and newsletters. These are the main "formal" sources from which speech-language pathologists and audiologists get the information they need to keep up to date. Many books are published every year that contain information that can be utilized by speech-language pathologists and audiologists. Some of these books are exhibited at professional conventions and/or are advertised in professional journals and newsletters. Speech-language

pathologists and audiologists are also alerted to the publication of new books by being mailed brochures and catalogues describing them. Another way that they are alerted to their availability is by joining a professional book club, such as the Library of Speech-Language Pathology. Such book clubs not only provide enrollees with information about new books, but they enable them to purchase books that are (or have been) main or alternative selections at a discount.

All professional associations distribute journals and/or newsletters to members. These publications both alert readers to new laws and other "realities" (e.g., those associated with the managed care philosophy) that may affect their scope of practice and provide useful information for coping with them. They may also alert readers to new opportunities, such as new grant programs.

- Viewing videotapes and listening to audiotapes. Videotapes and audiotapes are available for renting and/or purchase that illustrate diagnostic and treatment techniques. A developer of or advocate for a technique may be able to communicate it better to potential users by augmenting a written description of it with an audiotape and/or videotape. Many videotapes of this type have been presented at ASHA conventions. A list of these videotapes can be obtained from ASHA. ASHA also has audiotapes available of some its convention and workshop presentations. A listing of these audiotapes can also be obtained from ASHA.
- Interacting with tutorial software. There is interactive tutorial software available for both Windows and Macintosh computers that could be helpful to speech-language pathologists and audiologists. Some of it utilizes information from sites on the World Wide Web. And some of it is not intended solely for practitioners in our field (e.g., tutorials for word processing, database, and other general purpose computer software). While tutorial software was not a major continuing education source for our field when this chapter was written, it is likely to become one in the future.
- Doing treatment efficacy documentation (research). While doing treatment efficacy documentation (see Chapter 11) may not appear to be a continuing education activity, it can legitimately be regarded as being one. What you learn by doing such documentation can enable you to improve the efficacy of your treatments. And if you communicate what you learn by doing it to other clinicians, it can enable them to improve the efficacy of their treatments.

REFERENCES

Pietranton, A. A., & Lynch, C. (June/July, 1995). Multiskilling: A renaissance or a dark age? *Asha*, 37, 37–40.

Scope of practice in audiology (Spring, 1996). *Asha*, Supplement 16, 12–15.

Silverman, F. H. (1998). *Research Design and Evaluation in Speech-Language Pathology and Audiology* (4th ed.). Boston: Allyn & Bacon.

▶ 14

Being Culturally Sensitive

As a profession we are becoming increasingly aware of the ways that cultural diversity impacts on our functioning as clinicians. We now realize that performance on some diagnostic tests is significantly affected by cultural factors. Furthermore, we are becoming increasingly aware of the impacts that such factors can have on learning styles and the dynamics of the client-clinician relationship.

Before we begin our discussion of cultural considerations in managing communicative disorders, let's briefly consider what there is about culture that makes such considerations necessary. The following definition of culture by Porter and Samovar (1976, p. 7) provides some insight into this. They define culture as:

> *the cumulative deposit of knowledge, experience, meanings, beliefs, values, attitudes, religions, concepts of self, the universe, and self-universe relationships, hierarchies of status, role expectations, spatial relations, and time concepts acquired by a large group of people in the course of generations through individual and group striving. Culture manifests itself both in patterns of language and thought and in forms of activity and behavior. These patterns become models for common adaptive acts and styles of expressive behavior, which enable people to live in a society within a given geographical environment at a given state of technical development.*

Our focus in this chapter will be on some possible implications of these manifestations of culture and ethnicity for providing services to children and adults who have communicative disorders and their families. These implications will be discussed in the context of questions you should ponder before providing services to someone who has a cultural background different from your own. Your doing so can both facilitate your establishing a good clinical relationship with the person and his or her family and increase the likelihood that the assessment and treatment methods you use will be appropriate.

QUESTIONS TO PONDER

Manifestations of culture and ethnicity can make it necessary for you to function clinically somewhat differently than you would otherwise. By pondering the following questions before treating a client whose culture and ethnicity differs from yours, you are likely to become aware of at least some of the ways that it would be desirable for you to alter your clinical functioning.

- In what ways (if any) is it necessary for me to modify how I usually communicate verbally and nonverbally to avoid cultural taboos? Possible sources of such information about such taboos include books and articles about the culture, persons who are knowledgeable about the culture, and sites on the World Wide Web for persons who are visiting a country in which the client's cultural/ethnic group is a majority one.
- Are the stimuli in the diagnostic test(s) that I plan to use—particularly drawings and photographs—likely to elicit the same behaviors (responses) from persons in the client's culture as they are from persons in the culture in which the test was standardized? Some of the objects or events depicted may not be recognized by persons in the client's culture because they have not experienced them or they look different.
- Are the norms for the diagnostic test(s) I plan to use appropriate for persons having the client's cultural background? See Lahey (1992) and Seymour (1992) for discussions of several relevant issues.
- Are persons who have the client's cultural background as familiar with the tasks that the test(s) I will be using require them to do as the persons on whom the test was standardized? Lack of familiarity with how to perform a task can cause a test's standard instructions to be in-

sufficient, thereby making the accuracy of judgments based on its norms uncertain.

- Do persons having the client's cultural background tend to be as motivated to do well on the types of tests I will be administering as those in the culture in which the tests were standardized? Since motivation to do well affects test performance, the client's abilities are likely to be underestimated if this is not the case.

- Do language acquisition milestones tend to occur at the same ages in children in the client's culture as they do in the cultural groups on which the norms I will be using were based? This question can be particularly relevant for children who live (or have lived) in homes where English is not the language usually spoken. Their family could have lived in the United States for generations or be one that emigrated to the United States either before or after they were born.

- What questions (if any) should I add to and delete from the set that I usually ask when taking a case history to make it appropriate for a family from the client's culture? Some of the issues mentioned in this section (e.g., beliefs about causation) may suggest such questions.

- What habits, customs, values, and beliefs do persons having a particular cultural/ethnological background tend to hold or practice that could affect your relationship with the client and his or her family? Also, what attitudes toward expression of emotion and feelings, privacy, courtesy, respect for elders, behaviors related to family roles and sex roles, and the work ethic might they have that could affect this relationship?

- How important is it to families in the culture that children of the client's sex speak well? The amount of stress placed on speaking well in the culture may be different for girls than for boys.

- Does the client's communicative disorder call adverse attention to him or her in his or her culture? Differences in speech and language usage that may call adverse attention to a speaker in your culture may not do so in the client's culture. Conversely, some such differences that do not call adverse attention to a speaker in your culture may do so in the client's culture.

- What beliefs appear to be widely accepted by families in the client's culture about the etiology of communicative disorders? According to Anderson and Fenichel (1989), cultures differ markedly with regard to their beliefs about the etiology of disorders.

- From whom are the families in the client's culture likely to seek help for a person who has a communicative disorder—for example, a speech-language pathologist or audiologist, a physician, a chiropractor, a priest, a medicine man, an herbalist, an acupuncturist, a voodoo practitioner, a faith healer, a spiritualist, a minister? A practitioner other than a speech-language pathologist or audiologist would be likely to be consulted by families in some cultures for advice about treating a communicative disorder (Cole, 1989).

- What role (if any) in the client's culture do religious beliefs, sacred practices, or talismans tend to play in the treatment of disorders? Supernatural sources such as fate, evil spirits, or the punitive or retributive actions of a deity are regarded in some cultures as likely causes of disorders—including communicative disorders (Anderson & Fenichel, 1989; Fain, 1990; Maestas & Erickson, 1992; Wayman, Lynch, & Hanson, 1990).

- What beliefs appear to be widely accepted by families in the client's culture about the management of communicative disorders? In some cultures, for example, there is a belief that "a [communicative] disorder represents an act of God or demons and should not be tampered with" (Fain, 1990, p. 45).

- What beliefs appear to be widely accepted by families in the client's culture about factors that determine the efficacy of therapy? Bebout and Arthur (1992), for example, reported data that suggest that many Asians believe a willingness to "try hard" is the most important one.

- What stereotypes are there in the culture for persons who have the client's communicative disorder(s)? If there are no negative stereotypes, the disorder (or disorders) may not call adverse attention to the client and consequently, his or her motivation to invest in therapy may not be as great as it would be otherwise.

- How does having a communicative disorder like the client's tend to affect the self-concepts of persons in his or her culture? This would be determined, in part, by both what people in the culture believe to be its etiology and the impact that having it is likely to have on intelligence. If, for example, it was generally believed that the disorder is caused by "sin," the negative impact on self-concept is likely to be greater than it would tend to be if it was believed the disorder was caused by something that had nothing to do with the "moral status" of the client or his or her family. Likewise, if it was generally believed that the disorder caused a person to be less intelligent than they would have been otherwise, the negative impact on self-concept would tend to be greater than if there was no such belief.

- Does the client evince any communicative behaviors that are likely to call adverse attention to a speaker in his or her culture that would not tend to do so in yours? Such behaviors may relate to the pragmatics of communication. Since treatment efficacy is judged by a client's ability to communicate more effectively in his or her environment, it would probably be desirable to attempt to modify such behaviors if there are any.

- Does the type of therapeutic relationship that you usually establish with clients have to be modified in any way because of the client having a particular cultural background? If you are a male therapist treating an orthodox Moslem woman, you probably will have to modify your usual manner of interacting with clients at least a little. You are likely, for example, to have to allow one or more family members to be present in the therapy room during sessions.

- What stereotypes do you have about person's from the client's culture that could adversely affect your relationship with the client and his or her family? Almost everyone occasionally attributes undesirable personality traits to the members of some cultural/ethnic groups. Your tendency to attribute undesirable personality traits to persons in a client's cultural/ethnic group (assuming you do so) can adversely affect your relationship with him or her unless you are aware that your attributing them is based on a stereotype—not information that you have about the client.

- What alternative strategies can you devise for reducing the severity of the client's communicative disorder if the strategy of choice in your culture is not economically feasible? While the strategy of choice in your culture for augmenting the communication of persons with cerebral palsy who are severely speech impaired may be a computer-based, speech-generating communication aid, it may not be an option that is economically feasible in the client's culture. A cardboard communication board may be a more viable option. [Incidentally, research suggests that such a client will not necessarily communicate more effectively with a computerized device than he or she will with a cardboard communication board.]

- How might volunteers from the client's culture (under your supervision) be helpful in facilitating the management of his or her communicative disorder? They could, for example, serve as interpreters during sessions if the client didn't understand and/or speak English well.

- In what ways (if any) might members of the client's family be helpful in facilitating the management of the client's communicative disorder that ordinarily wouldn't be feasible in your culture? If, for example, it is common in the culture for grandparents to assume child-care responsibilities, it may be possible to utilize one or both of a child's grandparents for monitoring home assignments and reinforcing "new" communicative behaviors.

- What are the attitudes of persons in the client's cultural group toward seeking help? Doing so is widely regarded as "shameful" in some of them (Wayman, Lynch, & Hanson, 1990).

CULTURAL CONSIDERATIONS FOR TASK SELECTION

You have to take cultural factors into consideration when selecting tasks for answering questions if you want maximize the probability that your answers will be correct. An assessment task that yields data that are sufficiently valid and reliable for answering a particular question when administered to persons in your cultural/ethnic group may not do so when administered to persons in another. Performance on such tasks could be influenced by cultural factors in a number of ways, including the following:

- Some of the questions asked on "generic" case history forms may not be appropriate for persons who have a particular cultural background. Some questions that appear on such forms may not be relevant and others that are relevant do not appear. *Bloch's Ethnic/Cultural Assessment Guide* (Orque, Bloch, & Monroy, 1983) may be helpful to you when modifying such forms to make them culturally/ethnologically appropriate.

- Certain case history information obtained from informants (e.g., parents) may not be as accurate, complete, and/or appropriate for answering your questions as it would tend to be if obtained from persons in your culture. People differ in what they abstract and remember from what they observe—what they hear, see, smell, taste, and/or touch that they regard as significant and worth remembering.

Their "filters" are affected by manifestations of their culture and ethnicity, including their language (see Whorf, 1956). People tend to abstract things for which they have words and there are cultural differences in vocabulary, even among persons who speak the same language. There are also cultural differences in the meanings that particular words have for people. Consequently, your questions may not be interpreted as you expect them to be by informants whose culture and ethnicity differs from your own. And as a result of such breakdowns in communication, the information you obtain may be inaccurate or not as complete as you probably would assume it to be if it was provided by an informant who shared your culture and ethnicity. For information about structuring a case history interview to maximize the probability of getting accurate, relevant information from persons whose cultural background differs from yours, see Patton (1990, Chapter 7), Spradley (1979), Stewart and Cash (1988), and Taylor (1992).

- Persons having a client's cultural background and ethnicity may not be as familiar with a diagnostic task (particularly the stimuli used) as are the persons on whom its validity and reliability were established. If a client is less familiar with a task than those doing it are assumed to be, then his or her poor performance on the task could have resulted (at least in part) from a lack of familiarity with it rather than the deficit that the task was intended to detect. Some of the picture stimuli used in a language test, for example, may not be familiar to children having a certain cultural background; consequently, their inappropriate responses to such stimuli will not necessarily indicate that they have a language deficit.

- If a task is a test, the published norms may not be appropriate for persons having a client's (subject's) cultural background and ethnicity. There, of course, may not be any norms for a client's cultural/ethnic group available. Whenever the only norms available are ones for a cultural/ethnic group that is not a client's, conclusions and recommendations based on them should be made cautiously.

- A client's (subject's) motivation to do a particular task well may be influenced by his or her cultural background and ethnicity. We all have priorities that determine how well we have to do a task for us to be satisfied with our performance. While we have to do some tasks very well to satisfy ourselves, for others this is not the case. Our priorities are determined, in part, by the expected performance levels in our culture for the various tasks we are required to do. While earning high grades in school is a priority in some cultures, it is not so in others; consequently, children in the former are more likely to be motivated to achieve high grades than those in the latter. They are also more likely to be motivated to do well on diagnostic tasks than those in the latter.

- The language in which instructions and stimuli are communicated to a client or subject can affect his or her performance. If a client or subject is multilingual and the language used is not his or her first one, he or she may not perform as well as expected on a task because of a breakdown in communication. Also, if the instructions and/or stimuli for a task are translated from one language into another, performance may be affected by the translation not being equivalent to the original: It often is difficult to find words in two languages that convey exactly the same meaning.
- The sex and age of the clinician and the manner in which he or she interacts with the client may affect the client's performance. In some cultures, for example, males and females are not permitted to work together and consequently task performance may be affected by a person being uncomfortable working with someone of the opposite sex (Nellum-Davis, 1993).

It is crucial that when a cultural difference is observed in the performance on a task that *it not be interpreted as a deficit* (Cole, 1989; Martinez, Bedore, & Ludwig, 1994; Sue, 1983). You are particularly likely to do this if you use your culture as the "yardstick" for measuring other cultures. If persons from another culture tend to perform differently on a task (behavior) than they do in yours, this does not necessarily mean that their performance is less mature or inferior. The same, of course, is true for differences in attitude between persons from another culture and yours.

REFERENCES

Anderson, P., & Fenichel, E. (1989). *Serving Culturally Diverse Families of Infants and Toddlers with Disabilities*. Washington, DC: National Center for Clinical Infant Programs.

Bebout, L., & Arthur, B. (1992). Cross-cultural attitudes toward speech disorders. *Journal of Speech and Hearing Research, 35*, 45–52.

Cole, E. (1989). E pluribus pluribus: Multicultural imperatives for the 1990s and beyond. *Asha*, 31(9), 66–70.

Fain, M. (1990). Opportunities for service in third world countries. *Asha*, 32(5), 45–46.

Lahey, M. (1992). Linguistic and cultural diversity: Further problems for determining who shall be called language disordered. *Journal of Speech and Hearing Research*, 35, 638–639.

Maestas, A. G., & Erickson, J. G. (1992). Mexican immigrant mother's beliefs about disability. *American Journal of Speech-Language Pathology*, 1(4), 5–10.

Martinez, A., Bedore, L. M., & Ludwig, J. L. (1994). On cultural sensitivity in assessing cross-cultural attitudes: Comments on Bebout and Arthur (1992). *Journal of Speech and Hearing Research*, 37, 341–342.

Nellum-Davis, P. (1993). Clinical practice issues. In D. E. Battle (Ed.), *Communication Disorders in Multicultural Populations*. Boston: Andover Medical Publishers, 306–316.

Orque, M., Block, L., & Monroy, L. (1983). *Ethnic Nursing Care: A Multicultural Approach*. St. Louis, MO: C. V. Mosby.

Patton, M. Q. (1990). *Qualitative Evaluation and Research Methods*. Newbury Park, CA: Sage.

Porter, R. E., & Samovar, L. A. (1976). Communicating interculturally. In L. A. Samovar & R. W. Porter (Eds.), *Intercultural Education: A Reader*. Belmont, CA: Wadsworth.

Seymour, H. N. (1992). The invisible children: A reply to Lahey's perspective. *Journal of Speech and Hearing Research*, 35, 640–641.

Spradley, J. P. (1979). *The Ethnographic Interview*. New York: Holt, Rinehart, and Winston.

Stewart, C. J., & Cash, W. B. (1988). *Interviewing: Principles and Practices*. Dubuque, IA: William C. Brown.

Sue, S. (1983). Ethnic minority issues in psychology: A reexamination. *American Psychologist*, 38(5), 583–592.

Taylor, O. L. (1992). Clinical practice as a social occasion: An ethnographic model. In L. Cole & V. Deal (Eds.), *Communication Disorders in Multicultural Populations*. Rockville, MD: American Speech-Language-Hearing Association.

Wayman, I., Lynch, E., & Hanson, M. (1990). Home-based early childhood services: Cultural sensitivity in a family systems approach. *Topics in Early Childhood Special Education*, 10(4), 56–75.

Whorf, B. E. (1956). *Language, Thought, and Reality*. Cambridge, MA: Cambridge Technology Press of MIT.

▶ 15

Copyright Considerations for Clinicians

Speech-language pathologists and audiologists use various types of printed and audiovisual materials and computer software when functioning clinically. These include diagnostic tests, intervention programs, games, and photographs and drawings designed for eliciting speech and language samples, as well as computer software intended for meeting administrative responsibilities (e.g., word-processing software). Their use of these materials is regulated by copyright laws. These laws also protect the interests of practitioners who author materials of these types for clinical use. My objective in this chapter is to acquaint you with the aspects of copyright law that you need to know to both avoid breaking the law when utilizing clinical materials and to document your ownership of materials you create to facilitate your clinical activities.

OBJECTIVES OF COPYRIGHT LAW

Our government has recognized since its inception that authors should be allowed to profit from their creations. The source of this recognition appears to have been "natural law," which views it as only fair that authors be granted the exclusive right to benefit from their creations for a limited period of time. The framers of the Constitution, in fact, felt so strongly about the need to protect the right of authors to profit from their creations that they gave Congress the following power in Article 1, Section 8:

Congress shall have the power . . . to promote the progress of science and useful arts, by securing for limited times to authors and inventors the exclusive right to their respective writings and discoveries.

The mechanism that Congress created to protect the rights of authors was the copyright.

A copyright is the right to copy an author's work. The person owning the copyright, who may or may not be the author, has the *exclusive right* for a specified period of time to make and sell copies of the work; consequently, he or she holds the *copyright* for the work. The work may be perceivable by vision, audition, touch, or some combination of the three. Works of authorship that are perceivable by vision include books, computer programs, photographs, and drawings. An example of a work of authorship that is perceivable by audition is a "sound" recording on an audiotape cassette, computer disk, phonograph record, compact disk (CD), or digital audiotape (DAT) cartridge. And an example of a work of authorship that is perceivable by touch is a book printed in Braille. Examples of works of authorship that are perceivable through more than one sense modality are videotape recordings, sound motion pictures, and computer multimedia presentations.

Copyright laws have two basic objectives, both of which can be inferred from Article 1, Section 8 of the Constitution (quoted earlier in this chapter). The first "is to foster the creation and dissemination of intellectual works for the public welfare" (Dible, 1978, p. 115). These laws "foster the creation and dissemination of intellectual works" by giving the person who publishes them (who may or may not be their author) the opportunity to recoup expenses and possibly make a profit. They do this by making it unlawful for someone else to make copies of the work and sell them for the duration of its copyright. If there were no copyright laws, publishers would be hesitant to invest the money necessary to publish a work because someone else could make copies of the work and possibly sell them at a lower price since they would not have some of the production expenses of the original publisher such as copyediting and typesetting. (The assumption here is that they would copy the book photographically.)

The second objective of copyright laws "is to give the creators the *reward* [italics mine] due them for their contribution to society" (Dible, 1978, p. 115). They do this in two ways: first, by requiring anyone who copies part of an author's work to indicate the title of the work and the name of its author, and, second, by protecting the author's right to profit financially (e.g., by receiving royalties) from the sale of copies of his or her works. No one is permitted to make and sell copies of an author's work without permission for the duration of the copyright. Presumably, if an author gives someone permission to make and sell copies of a work that he or she created, the author will be paid a certain agreed to amount for the permission to do so (possibly as a royalty on each copy sold).

PROVISIONS OF COPYRIGHT LAW

The regulations pertaining to copyrights in the United States are contained in the Copyright Act of 1976 (Public Law 94-553). This was the first general revision of U.S. copyright law since 1909. The act became fully effective on January 1, 1978.

The Copyright Act of 1976 is a complex statute. Because of space limitations, I cannot discuss all aspects (or even all major aspects) of it here. My presentation will be limited to aspects that are likely to be relevant to the activities of speech-language pathologists and audiologists. The order in which topics are discussed corresponds roughly to the order in which they are mentioned in the statute. (The primary source for this discussion was Dible, 1978, pp. 111–254.)

Duration of Copyright Protection

For works of authorship created after January 1, 1978, the duration of copyright protection is the life of the author plus fifty years after his or her death. For works of more than one author, the fifty-year period is measured from the date of the death of the last surviving author. All copyrights run through December 31 of the calendar year in which they expire.

Material That Can Be Copyrighted

The 1976 Copyright Act substitutes the phrase "original works of authorship" for "writings of an author" when designating the material that can be copyrighted. Original works of authorship that can be copyrighted under this act are not limited to those containing written words (which are referred to in the statute as "literary works"). These also include: (1)

pictorial, graphic, and sculptural works, (2) motion pictures and other audiovisual works, (3) sound recordings, and (4) computer programs.

The category of *literary works* includes any works expressed in "words, numbers, or other verbal or numerical symbols or indicia." While a literary work has to be original in the sense of not being merely a copy of a preexisting work, there is no requirement that it be novel, or ingenuous, or possess esthetic merit. Almost any diagnostic or progress report could be classified for purposes of copyright as a "literary work."

The category of *pictorial, graphic, and sculptural works* includes photographs and drawings (such as those used in diagnostic tests and kits of therapy materials). Photographs and drawings, like literary works, must be original in the sense of not being merely copies of preexisting images, but their novelty, ingenuity, or esthetic merit are not considerations in determining whether they can be copyrighted.

The category of *motion pictures and other audiovisual works* includes videotapes (e.g., videotapes of diagnostic and therapy sessions made by clinicians); the category of *sound recordings* includes phonograph records, audiotapes (e.g., speech and language samples recorded for clinical purposes), compact disks (CDs), and digital audiotape (DAT) cartridges. Again, novelty, ingenuity, or esthetic merit are not considerations in determining whether a work can be copyrighted.

The category of *computer programs* includes both the code of which programs are comprised and the audiovisual displays that the code produces. These may be copyrighted separately because substantially the same visual and/or audiovisual effect can be achieved by different sets of computer code (Chickering & Hartman, 1987). With computer programs (as with the other categories of material) novelty, ingenuity, or esthetic merit are not considerations in determining whether a work can be copyrighted.

Thus far in this section I have dealt with material that can be copyrighted. What *cannot* be copyrighted? There are six types of materials mentioned in the act that are denied U.S. copyright protection. Three are likely to be of particular interest to speech-language pathologists and audiologists. The first of these is *ideas, methods, systems, and principles*. One of the fundamental principles promulgated by this act is that "copyright does not protect ideas, methods, systems, principles, etc. but rather the *particular manner* [italics mine] in which they are expressed or described" (Dible, 1978, p. 127). Consequently, a copyright does not protect a clinician's ideas or methods from being copied; it only protects the particular arrangement of words in which he or she expresses or describes them.

A second type of subject matter that is denied U.S. copyright protection is *blank forms*. According to Dible (1978, p. 127), "Blank forms and similar works designed to record rather than convey information, are not subject to copyright protection." Some of the forms used for recording client's responses to diagnostic tests probably are not protected by copyright for this reason, even though a copyright notice is printed on them. Anyone can place a copyright notice on any work he or she creates, including material that cannot be copyrighted. The copyright notice on such an uncopyrightable test form does serve to discourage others from copying it, simply because most people who use it are not sufficiently familiar with copyright law to know that it cannot be copyrighted.

A third type of subject matter that is denied U.S. copyright protection is *works of the U.S. Government*. According to Dible (1978, p. 128), "works produced for the U.S. Government by its officers and employees *as a part of their official duties* [italics mine] are not subject to U.S. copyright protection." This category does not necessarily include works prepared under a U.S. government contract or grant. The funding agency can decide whether an independent contractor or grantee will be allowed to copyright works that were supported wholly or partially by government funds.

Ownership and Transfer of Rights

The author of a work that was not prepared within the scope of his or her employment is the owner of the copyright on it unless he or she has transferred ownership of the copyright to somebody else. If such a work has more than one author, its authors jointly own the copyright unless they have transferred ownership of the copyright to somebody else.

The copyright to a "work prepared by an employee within the scope of his or her employment" belongs to the employer unless the employer transfers it to the employee in writing. Such a work is referred to in the Copyright Act as a *work made for hire*. "The rationale for this rule is that the work is produced under the employer's direction and expense; also the employer bears the risks and should be allowed to reap the benefits" (Dible, 1978, p. 130). Your employer, however, would not be entitled to the copyright on a work you authored that was not prepared within the scope of your employment. If you plan to author something from which you hope to profit financially and if you will be doing it wholly or partially on the job and/or at your employer's expense, your employer may feel that he or she will be entitled to ownership of the copyright on it. To avoid a misunderstanding when the "work" is completed, it probably would be a good idea before beginning it to request a letter from your employer acknowledging your right to copyright the work in your name (or if your employer contributes significantly to the creation of it, in both your names). Another way to avoid such a misunderstanding is to work on the project at home on your own time.

Why might an author wish to transfer his or her rights to a work to somebody else? The reason in most cases would be that the author expected to profit from doing so. A publisher, for example, may agree to pay the author a royalty on each copy of his work sold in exchange for this transfer of rights. An author can sometimes negotiate a contract that allows him or her to retain the copyright on a work and then only sell (usually through an agent) certain rights to publishers (e.g., translation rights). By negotiating this type of contract the author is in effect transferring ownership of a part of the copyright.

Reproduction of Copyrighted Materials and the Doctrine of Fair Use

The Copyright Act of 1976 places certain restrictions on prohibiting the reproduction of copyrighted materials. On such restriction has been referred to as the *doctrine of fair use*. For an in-depth discussion of this doctrine, see the Copyright Act and Dible (1978).

The doctrine of fair use, which was developed by the courts, "allows copying without permission from, or payment to, the copyright owner where the use is reasonable and not harmful to the rights of the copyright owner" (Dible, 1978, p. 142). Without this doctrine, no use of copyrighted material would be possible without the copyright owner's permission. The idea here is that certain uses of copyrighted materials are not harmful to the rights of the copyright owner and promote the *public welfare*.

What can be copied under this doctrine? The excerpt from Section 107 of the Act, reproduced below, though somewhat vague, provides some general guidelines:

> . . . *the fair use of a copyrighted work, including such use by reproduction in copies or phonograph records or by other means . . . for purposes*

such as criticism, comment, news reporting, teaching (including multiple copies for classroom use), scholarship, or research, is not an infringement of copyright. In determining whether the use made of a work in any particular case is a fair use the factors to be considered shall include—

1. *the purpose and character of the use, including whether such use is of a commercial nature or is for nonprofit educational purposes;*
2. *the nature of the copyrighted work;*
3. *the amount and substantiality of the portion used in relation to the copyrighted work as a whole; and*
4. *the effect of the use upon the potential market for or value of the copyrighted work.*

In addition to these general guidelines for applying the fair use doctrine, specific ones have been developed for several areas. One such area is teaching. These guidelines permit teachers to make *single copies* of copyrighted materials for use in their teaching. They also permit teachers to make *multiple copies* for classroom use if the number of copies does not exceed the number of pupils in the class and the following restrictions are adhered to:

1. *the copies may not be used as a substitute for anthologies, compilations, or collective works;*
2. *copies cannot be made of consumable materials such as workbooks;*
3. *the copies cannot be a substitute for purchases, be "directed by higher authority," or be repeated by the same teacher from term to term; and*
4. *there is no charge to the student beyond the actual copying cost. (Dible, 1978, p. 143)*

Notice of Copyright

It is *desirable* that a copyright notice be placed on all works for which copyright protection is desired. On visually perceptible copies, the notice should contain the following three elements:

1. *the symbol © (the letter c in a circle), or the word "Copyright," or the abbreviation "Copr.";*

2. *the year of the first publication of the work; and*
3. *the name of the owner of the copyright in the work, or an abbreviation by which the name can be recognized, or a generally known designation of the owner. (Dible, 1978, pp. 228–229)*

However, "subject to certain safeguards for innocent infringers, protection would not be lost by the complete omission of the notice from large numbers of copies or from a whole edition, if registration of the work is made before or within *five years after publication* [italics mine]" (Dible, 1978, p. 165). Consequently, immediate, formal application for a copyright is not a prerequisite for placing a copyright notice on a work or for securing copyright protection for it. The mere placement of a copyright notice on a work ordinarily is sufficient to discourage persons from copying it without permission. The formal registration of a copyright, however, does increase the number of types of remedies that its owner can seek from a court.

Deposit and Registration of the Work for Which Copyright Protection Is Sought

The formal copyrighting of a work ordinarily involves (1) depositing two complete copies in the Library of Congress and (2) completing an application for copyright registration and paying the required fee. (For an in-depth description of the application procedure, see Chickering & Hartman, 1987.) Depositing the two copies of the work in the Library of Congress isn't always a prerequisite for securing copyright protection. It would not be one if fewer than five copies of the work have been published or the work is an expensive limited edition with numbered copies for which the requirement to deposit two copies would be burdensome, unfair, or unreasonable (see Section 407C of the 1976 Copyright Act). A slide-tape presentation or a videotape production that a speech-language pathologist or audiologist publishes in a limited edition *may* be exempt from the deposit requirement.

Copyright Infringement and Remedies

Owners of a copyright can seek several types of remedies from a court if the copyright is infringed. They can ask the court to issue an *injunction or restraining order* that will temporarily or permanently prevent or stop infringements. They can ask the court to *impound* all allegedly infringing copies of the work during the time a suit for infringement is pending. They can ask the court to award *compensatory damages* that would offset the profits they lost because of the sale of the infringer's copies. Or they can ask the court to award them *statutory damages,* which are a type of punitive damages that defendants can be required to pay simply because they infringed the plaintiff's copyright. They are referred to as *statutory damages* because they are specified in the statute, or law.

REFERENCES

Chickering, R. B., & Hartman, M S. (1987). *How to Register a Copyright and Protect Your Creative Work.* New York: Charles Scribner's Sons.

Dible, D. M. (Ed.) (1978). *What Everybody Should Know About Patents, Trademarks, and Copyrights.* Fairfield, CA: Entrepreneur Press.

▶ 16

Legal and Tax Implications of Employment Relationships

Your role while meeting your responsibilities as a speech-language pathologist or audiologist may be what the courts refers to as that of a master, a servant, a principal, an agent, an independent contractor, an employer, or some combination of these. If you are receiving money for your services, your role could be that of a servant, an agent, or an independent contractor. If you contract for and/or supervise the services of others, your role could be that of a master, a principal, or an employer. And if you both receive a salary and are involved in the hiring and/or supervision of other persons, your role would be a combination of them. Three combinations of these role definitions are used by the courts when deciding cases concerning the responsibilities of employers to employees and supervisors to supervisees. Certain of these definitions are also used by state and federal governments for defining tax liability. Some legal and tax implications of these roles and relationships are explored in this chapter.

MASTER–SERVANT, PRINCIPAL–AGENT, AND EMPLOYER–INDEPENDENT CONTRACTOR RELATIONSHIPS

The specific legal responsibilities of an employer to an employee and of an employee to an employer depend on whether their relationship would be viewed by the courts as being that of a *master to a servant*, a *principal to an agent,* or an *employer to an independent contractor.* Your legal responsibilities and liabilities as an employee in a particular situation are determined by whether in that situation you are functioning as a "servant," an "agent," or an "independent contractor." Your relationship to an employer or to the person, or persons, who assign you responsibilities may be that of a servant to a master under some circumstances. Under others it may be that of an agent to a principal or an independent contractor to an employer. The terms "master" and "servant" are used metaphorically in this context.

One of the main differences among these three types of relationships is the amount of responsibility that one person assumes for the activities of the other. The employer/supervisor assumes more such responsibility in the master–servant relationship than in the principal–agent one. He or she assumes least responsibility for the other's activities in the employer–independent contractor relationship.

What are the characteristics of a *master–servant relationship*? According to Black:

> *The relationship of master and servant exists where one person, for pay or other valuable consideration [e.g., "hours" toward satisfying a clinical practicum requirement] enters into the service of another and devotes to him his personal labor for an agreed period . . . It usually contemplates employer's right to* prescribe *[emphasis mine] end and direct means and method of doing work. (1968, p. 1127)*

Consequently, in this type of relationship the employer/supervisor prescribes not only *what* the other is to do, but *how* he or she is to do it.

The relationship between a speech-language pathologist and a speech-language pathology assistant would be a master–servant one. The relationship between a speech-language pathologist or audiologist functioning as a practicum supervisor and a student clinician would also be of this type.

Because an employee in a master–servant relationship theoretically is following orders, the person giving the orders (e.g., the person prescribing therapy) is legally responsible for any damage done to person or property by the employee that resulted from the orders being carried out. This is referred to as *vicarious liability* because the person who does the "deed" is not the one who has to assume responsibility for it (Woody, 1986). Physicians have traditionally had relationships of this type with nurses, physical therapists, occupational therapists, and other health professionals who deliver services that physicians prescribe. Some relatively recent court decisions, however, have held such persons partially responsible for damage done to patients as a consequence of a prescription being carried out. Health-care paraprofessionals are particularly likely to be expected to share responsibility for such damage if they are aware that a prescribed treatment they are administering to a patient is likely to be harmful.

What are the characteristics of a *principal–agent relationship*? According to Black, an agent is

> *one who deals not only with things, as does a servant, but with persons,* using his own discretion as to means *[emphasis mine], and frequently establishes contractual relations between his principal and third persons. (1968, pp. 85–86)*

An "agent," therefore, differs from a "servant" in the following two ways: First, an agent ordinarily is not told specifically how to carry out assigned duties, but is permitted to use "his own discretion as to means." For example, a speech-language pathologist employed by a school system who is functioning in this role would be told to provide clinical services to children at a particular school, but the particular children he or she served and how he or she served them would be left to his or her own discretion.

A second way in which an agent differs from a servant is that agents can *establish contractual relations* between their employer (i.e., principal) and third persons. For example, a public-school speech-language pathologist would be establishing a contractual relationship between her employer and a particular test publisher (third person) when she ordered a diagnostic test from that publisher for use in her school—that is, she would be obligating her employer to pay for the test.

Speech-language pathologists and audiologists who are employed by schools, hospitals, or other institutions ordinarily function as agents. Consequently, they have to assume some legal responsibility for any damage they do to their clients. They probably would not have to assume the full responsibility if they committed a tort because a court would be likely to view the employer (principal) as tacitly certifying their professionalism and competence by employing them. Consequently, an employer probably would have to assume some of responsibility for any damage that a clinician did to a client.

What are the characteristics of an *employer–independent contractor relationship*? According to Black, an independent contractor is

> *one who, exercising an independent employment, contracts to do a piece of work according to his own methods and without being subject to the control of his employer except as to the results of the work.* (1968, p. 911)

Consequently, "independent contractors" differ from "agents" and "servants" in several ways. First, they are self-employed. They contract with their employers to do a particular piece of work. An audiologist, for example, might contract with an industrial firm to screen its employees for noise-induced hearing loss for an agreed-upon fee per employee. The audiologist would not be an employee of the firm. He or she would be a self-employed professional who was paid a fee to perform "a piece of work" (i.e., a hearing screening). After the hearing tests were administered and the results reported, his or her relationship with the firm would end.

A second way that independent contractors differ from agents and servants (particularly the latter) is that their employers ordinarily do not specify how the work is to be performed. They specify the desired results in the contract and ordinarily leave the means to the discretion of the independent contractor. The audiologist in our previous example to fulfill the contract would have to report the status of each employee's hearing to the firm. He or she could use any audiometric testing procedure that would be expected to yield data possessing adequate levels of validity and reliability.

A third way that independent contractors differ from agents and servants is that they have to assume full responsibility for any damage that they do. Speech-language pathologists and audiologists in private practice are independent contractors. As such, they have to assume full responsibility for any harm they bring about. They would be wise, therefore, to purchase professional liability insurance. Information about companies that sell such insurance can be obtained from the American Speech-Language-Hearing Association.

Thus far, we have considered the employer–employee relationship primarily from the perspective of the employee. When we consider the role of the employee as a servant, agent, or independent contractor from an *employer's perspective*, one of the main concerns is the employer's responsibility for his or her employees' work-related torts and broken (breached) contracts. The concept that one person can be held responsible for another person's torts and broken contracts is referred to in the legal literature as the doctrine of *respondeat superior*. "The fundamental rule generally recognized is that the doctrine of *respondeat superior* is applicable to the relation of master and servant or of principal and agent, but not to that of employer and independent contractor" (from court opinion in *Miller v. Metropolitan Live Insurance Company, 134 Ohio St. 289*). Consequently, employers can protect themselves from responsibility for the work-related torts and broken contracts of their employees by utilizing independent contractors. A nursing home, for example, probably could protect itself from tort litigation associated with the delivery of speech, language, and hearing services by contracting with a private practitioner for their delivery.

GOVERNMENT REGULATION OF THE EMPLOYER–EMPLOYEE RELATIONSHIP

Many aspects of the employer–employee relationship are regulated directly or indirectly by either the state or federal government, including the following:

- Factors to consider when deciding whether to hire, fire, or promote someone
- The nature of the physical work environment
- The manner in which employer–employee disputes are resolved
- The compensation of employees for their services

Some implications of each of these are indicated in the following paragraphs.

An employer ordinarily is not permitted to hire, fire, or promote employees strictly on the basis of whether he or she likes them. A number of laws prohibit discrimination in hiring and promotion on the basis of extraneous (to the requirements of the job) employee characteristics such as age, gender, race, religion, sexual orientation, and/or possession of a disability. Some regulations go one step further. They require preference to be given in hiring and promotion to persons against whom society has discriminated in the past. This is referred to as *affirmative action*.

The government also regulates to some extent the conditions under which work is performed. The main thrust of government regulation in this area appears to be the minimizing of hazards to workers' health. One federal administrative agency that is quite involved with this area is the Occupational Safety and Health Administration (OSHA). An example of an aspect of the work environment that OSHA has attempted to regulate is ambient noise level.

The government has also made some attempt to regulate how disputes between employers and employees are resolved. Persons associated with government agencies have been instrumental in arbitrating such disputes. The government is unlikely to do so, however, unless a dispute is viewed as seriously threatening the public interest.

Many government regulations deal with how employees are to be compensated for their services. They deal with such matters as the minimum wage that can be offered an employee, employers' and employees' contributions to employees' social security accounts, and the percentages of wages that must be withheld for state and federal income taxes.

TAX IMPLICATIONS OF EMPLOYER–INDEPENDENT CONTRACTOR RELATIONSHIP

If your relationship to an employer is that of an independent contractor, social security and income tax will not be withheld from your check nor will you receive any benefits, including malpractice insurance. The government, including the IRS, will regard you as operating a small business. Consequently, you will be expected to keep the kinds of tax records that all small businesses are required to keep and to make quarterly payments to the IRS if more than a certain percentage of your income is from this source. You will be a full- or part-time private practitioner whether or not you intended to be one.

A speech-language pathologist or audiologist could become an independent contractor without intending to become one. If, for example, you accepted a part-time job at a nursing home for a certain amount an hour and nothing was withheld from your first check, your status there would probably be that of an independent contractor. If you do not want to operate a small business (i.e., be an private practitioner), you should inquire whether your relationship to your employer will be that of an agent or an independent contractor before accepting a part-time job.

Your working as an independent contractor is not necessarily disadvantageous from the tax point of view. You will be allowed certain deductions that you wouldn't be otherwise. For example, you will be allowed to deduct the cost of transportation (e.g., car mileage) to and from where you are working. Before accepting a position where your status will be that of an independent contractor, you would be wise to discuss the tax implications of your doing so with a CPA.

REFERENCES

Black, H. C. (1968). *Black's Law Dictionary* (Rev. 4th ed.). St. Paul, MN: West Publishing Company.

Woody, R. H. (1986). Legal issues for private practitioners in speech-language pathology and audiology. In K. G. Butler (Ed.), *Prospering in Private Practice*. Rockville, MD: Aspen.

▶ 17

Templates and Other Strategies for Facilitating Clinical Report Writing

Part of your responsibility as a speech-language pathologist or audiologist is to write reports, including evaluation and progress reports. Doing so can be very time consuming and is unlikely to be one of your favorite activities. Assuming that you are using a computer with word-processing software for report writing, there are several strategies you can use that are likely to reduce the time it takes you to draft at least some reports. In addition to saving time, the use of these strategies may enable you to produce reports that communicate information more clearly and contain fewer grammatical and other errors. These strategies are described in this chapter.

TEMPLATES

The majority of your evaluation and progress reports are likely to have a standard format. Your evaluation reports, for example, are likely to begin with certain identifying information, including the client's name and address. When writing such a report you would keyboard both the headings (NAME, ADDRESS) and the identifying information.

Some of the sentences and paragraphs that appear in your evaluation reports for a particular disorder are likely to be either the same or the same except for blanks. An example of a sentence containing blanks is the following: "The client's air conduction threshold in the left ear at 1000 Hz was _____ dB." Almost all of the sentences and paragraphs in some types of evaluation reports (those for routine audiometric tests) are either the same or the same expect for blanks.

Even sentences and paragraphs that you use for presenting test results in such reports are likely to be similar. For example, an pure-tone audiometric screening test can have two possible outcomes—that is, the test was passed at all frequencies or the test was failed at one or more frequencies. The sentence or group of sentences that you routinely use to report and interpret each of these outcomes are likely to be similar.

Some of the sentences and paragraphs that you use routinely in progress reports are also likely to be standard ones. However, you may not use as many standard sentences and paragraphs in progress reports as you do in evaluation ones.

When you use a standard sentence or paragraph in a report you have to keyboard it. Doing so both takes time and increases the possibility for error. One way to minimize both is to create a template for the report. A template is a word-processor file. A template for a report for a particular type of hearing test, for example, would be a word-processor file that contained all of the standard sentences and paragraphs that could appear in the report arranged appropriately. Some sentences would contain blanks (e.g., for reporting thresholds) and there may be several alternative recommendation paragraphs—one for each outcome that occurs frequently.

To create a template for a particular report, you would keyboard the standard sentences and paragraphs in the way you want them to appear in the report. You would save the resulting word-processor file either in the usual way or in a "stationary" format. If you saved it in the usual way, you would lock it (i.e., designate it as "read only"). If you save it in a stationary format (which is preferable if your word-processing program has this option), it will be locked automatically. Incidentally, you can modify a template by unlocking it, making your changes, and then relocking it.

To write a report using a template, you would open the file for it. You would then fill in the blanks, delete any sentences and/or paragraphs you don't want to include, make any necessary modifications to the "boilerplate" text in it, and add any additional sentences or paragraphs that are needed. You would then save the resulting report as you would any word-processor file. The reason for locking the template file is to keep it from being deleted accidentally from your diskette or hard disk. This would happen if a template's file format was not a stationary one and you saved a report as you usually do. To save a report for which you used a template you would use your word-processor's "save as" (or equivalent) command.

One strategy for insuring that all of the blanks in a report introduced by using a template will be filled in is to designate the location of each blank in the template with a series of three Xs (XXX). You would use your word-processor's "find" command to locate the first blank (i.e., XXX), delete the Xs, and fill it in. You would then issue the "find" command again (to locate the second blank), delete the Xs, and fill it in. You would keep repeating this process until all of the blanks have been filled in.

The sentences and paragraphs that you include in the template could come from reports that you have drafted and/or from ones drafted by others. See Appendix A of Silverman (1996) for some sentences and paragraphs that could be used in a template for a fluency evaluation report.

PRINT (MAIL) MERGE UTILITIES

A print (mail) merge utility merges the contents of two files when printing a document. One is likely to be a word-processor file and the other a database file. The resulting document contains text from both. This is the type of utility that is used for printing form letters.

If you have client information (e.g., name, address, and telephone number) in a database file that you want to include in a report for which you are using a template, you can include instructions in the template file that will automatically cause the computer to merge the information from the database into the template file when the report is printed. Using this strategy would both save time (less keyboarding would be necessary) and reduce the likelihood that the information merged (e.g., names and addresses) would be spelled incorrectly. See your word-processor's manual for information on how to use its merge utility.

MACROS

If there is certain information that you include in many of your reports (such as your name and address), you can create a macro that will keyboard it for you. A macro is a recording of a series of keystrokes and/or mouse movements that is "played" whenever you press a particular key or key combination (e.g., control-A). Macros can also facilitate your report writing in other ways, including the following:

- Copy the inside address from a cover letter and print it on an envelope or address label
- Transmit a copy of a report to a fax machine or a computer that has been programmed to simulate one
- Transmit a copy of a report to an e-mail address

ABBREVIATION-EXPANDING UTILITIES

These utilities can enable you to type the multisyllable technical terms, phrases, sentences, and paragraphs that you include frequently in reports by keyboarding a three- or four-letter abbreviation and then pressing a key (e.g., the space bar) that causes the abbreviation to expand. Keyboarding "bsn" and pressing the space bar, for example, could cause the computer to delete "bsn" from the monitor screen and replace it with the phrase "bilateral sensorineural hearing loss." You can keyboard any word, phrase, sentence, or paragraph in this manner and choose the abbreviation for it. The maximum number of abbreviations that the software will recognize is likely to be in the hundreds. By using this type of utility, you can both keyboard reports a little faster and reduce the likelihood of typos, particularly on technical terms. [The utility of this type that I use, incidentally, is the Macintosh shareware one *TypeIt4Me*.]

SPELLING CHECKERS

Your word-processing software probably has a spell-check utility built in. Even if you're an expert typist, you will occasionally make errors. The fastest and surest way for you to identify and correct typos and spelling errors in a report is to use the software's spell-check utility. Its dictionary is unlikely to contain all of the technical terms that you use in reports routinely. You can reduce the length of time it will take to spell-check future reports by adding the terms the software flags that are spelled correctly to the utility's custom dictionary.

GRAMMAR CHECKERS

These utilities identify errors in grammar, punctuation, usage, style, and spelling and offer suggestions for correcting them. Current versions of some word-processing programs (including Microsoft Word) have a grammar-check utility. The types of grammatical and stylistic errors that they can identify include the following:

- Subject-verb agreement
- Pronoun errors
- Clause errors
- Punctuation errors
- Spelling errors
- Inappropriate prepositions
- Split infinitives
- Clichés
- Vague qualifiers
- Multiple negation
- Misused words
- Overused phrases

These utilities can be set to ignore certain types of errors. Since grammar-check utilities can also identify misspelled words, it is not necessary to use a spell-check utility on a report if you will be using a grammar-check utility when editing it.

Most grammar-check utilities also assess the "readability" of a document. They automatically compute a reading grade level index for it, such as the Flesch index. This information can be crucial when drafting reports and other documents (e.g., consent forms) for clients and/or their families. It is particularly likely to be useful if their reading grade level for English is fairly low.

The routine use of a grammar-check utility can enhance the professionalism, clarity, and readability of your clinical reports. Some of the types of "errors" that the software flags may not really be errors but aspects of your writing style that do not detract for the professionalism, clarity, or readability of your reports. By modifying the software's preference file to stop it from flagging these types of "errors, " you can both speed up the checking process and reduce your frustration while using the utility.

THESAURUS UTILITIES

Your word-processing software is likely to have a thesaurus utility that will display synonyms for a word you "highlight" and replace that word with one of the synonyms it displays if you tell it to do so. Thesaurus utility programs are also available that are fully compatible with Microsoft Word and other word-processing programs and contain a larger number of synonyms. [The Macintosh one that I use is *Big Thesaurus*.] The routine use of these utilities can improve clarity of your reports. When you edit a report and come across a word that you feel doesn't quite convey your meaning, you can use the utility to search for a better synonym.

PERSONAL DIGITAL ASSISTANTS AND LAPTOP COMPUTERS

If you take notes while testing and/or taking a case history with a laptop computer or personal digital assistant, you can transfer them to the report. You can do so manually by "cutting" them from the note file and "pasting" them in the report at appropriate locations. You may also be able to do so automatically using a print merge utility (these are described elsewhere in the chapter). To do so, you would create a form that would be displayed on the screen of the laptop computer or personal digital assistant and filled in by you. Codes for the items on the form would be inserted into the template you are using to write the report. The print merge utility would copy information from the file created by the laptop computer or personal digital assistant and "paste" it into the report where the codes indicate it should be inserted. "Pasting" information into a report in one of these two ways both reduces the amount of keyboarding that you have to do and eliminates a source of error, the typos when keyboarding the report.

REFERENCES

Silverman, F. H. (1996). *Stuttering and Other Fluency Disorders* (2nd ed.). Boston: Allyn & Bacon.

Index